27 WAYS TO INCREASE YOUR CHILD'S IQ

And Unleash the Genius Within

By

Jagir S. Reehal, PH.D.

Website: www.thesuccessfulkid.com

ISBN 978-1-78555-037-9

Published by
Inspired Publishing Books
Inspired Publishing Ltd
27 Old Gloucester Street
London WC1N 3AX

DEDICATION

"Children make your life important."

— Erma Bombeck, American humourist

This book is dedicated to my children

CONTENTS

Who This Book Is For

The information in this book will be valuable to the following:

- Couples who are planning to have children or already have children.

- Grandparents who want to help to improve the IQ score of their grandchildren.

- People of all ages who have an interest in improving their IQ.

Many of the strategies presented in this book are not age-specific and can be used by anyone.

How to Read the Book

The book is composed of 27 small chapters grouped into four sections: Pre-conception, Pregnancy and Parents; Early Years and Beyond; Nutrition Diet and Health; Additional Tips. In some cases, there is a slight degree of overlap. This is necessary to contextualise some chapters or paragraphs.

There is no set way to read this book. Each chapter is a standalone chapter, so you can read it from cover to cover or cherry-pick certain chapters.

PREFACE

"Children are one third of our population and all of our future."

— *Select Panel for the Promotion of Child Health, 1981*

What is IQ?

IQ is short for Intelligence Quotient. The IQ score is a relative measure that compares the abilities of people of the **same age**. What an IQ test measures is not actual intelligence, but a person's *capacity for intelligence* – that is, the IQ test measures a person's ability to learn information.

Modern IQ tests produce scores for different areas such as language fluency and three-dimensional thinking, and the overall score is calculated from subtest scores.

There are many different types of IQ tests and each has its own scale, however, they all agree that an IQ score of around 100 is a person of average intelligence. Anything above 100 is considered as above average and under 100 is below average. An IQ score below 70 is taken as that of mentally-challenged person. An IQ score above 140 is generally considered as that of a genius.

The IQ of some famous people

Christopher Hirata	Astrophysicist	225
Leonardo Da Vinci	Poet/Writer/Genius	220
Goethe	Poet/Writer/Genius	210
Emanuel Swedenborg	Religious writer/Genius	205
Leibniz	Philosopher/Mathematician	205
Blaise Pascal	Mathematician/Physicist	195

JAGIR S. REEHAL, PH.D.

Sir Isaac Newton	Mathematician/Scientist	190
Bobby Fischer	Chess player	187
Galileo Galilei	Physicist/Astronomer/Philosopher	185
René Descartes	Philosopher/Mathematician	180
Immanuel Kant	Philosopher	175
Mozart	Composer	165
Albert Einstein	Mathematician/Physicist	161
George Eliot	Writer	160
Stephen Hawking	Scientist	160
Thomas Edison	Writer	150
Madonna	Musician	140
Barrack Obama	President	130
John F. Kennedy	President	119
George Bush Sr	President	98
Andy Warhol	Artist	86
Muhammad Ali	Boxer	78

What are the components of an IQ test?

Logical reasoning, problem solving, critical thinking, and adaptation are all important components of intelligence. An IQ test, therefore, must necessarily evaluate a candidate's abilities in all the following areas:

- Verbal intelligence
- Mathematical ability
- Spatial reasoning skills
- Visual/perceptual skills
- Classification skills
- Logical reasoning skills
- Pattern recognition skills

In addition to these intellectual skills, life situations are considered through psychological and sociological tests.

However, IQ tests do not, as yet, measure creativity, musical affinity, intrinsic motivation, spiritual gifts, non-academic talents, musical abilities, manual dexterity, interpersonal skills, and similar skills.

How to measure your child's IQ

To measure your child's IQ, you can do one of several IQ tests online — just search the internet for "online IQ test". However, if you want your child to be eligible to join one of the high IQ societies such as Mensa, then an online test will not be enough. You must contact the organisation concerned to sit one of their standardised IQ tests.

Why you should act on the information in this book

1. **It will help you to understand your child:** One of the most important reasons to have your children tested is to gain an insight into their strengths and weaknesses. Test scores give parents valuable information about a child's potential. Just as a child who has a low IQ may face problems at school, for a gifted child, school may be so boring that they develop mental and behavioural issues, which may lead to unnecessary, and occasionally tragic, outcomes.

    In his book *Tools of Titans*, Tim Ferris writes, *"Humans are imperfect creatures. You don't "succeed" because you have no weaknesses; you "succeed" because you find your unique strengths and focus on developing habits around them."*

    The results of an IQ test along with other information can help to identify your child's unique strengths and enable you to focus on developing these strengths rather than being critical of their weaknesses.

2. **You child will have an advantage:** A high IQ is a powerful asset in today's knowledge-based economy and pays off in terms of increased income and professional success. In today's competitive world, people who can absorb and process knowledge fast stand

a better chance of winning. The more complex life becomes, the more advantageous it becomes to have a high IQ. In a complex and technically advanced society, a high IQ is an asset, but a superior IQ will be advantage.

3. **Your child will become more resilient:** A high IQ helps to make children more resilient in early life. The 1998 National Study of Youth looked at the well-being of 466 children. Within this sample group, the researcher Jody Hendrix found some children who were, as she defined them, "resilient". These children showed no signs of depression, delinquency, or school failure. Upon analysis, she identified that the 160 most resilient children tended to have the highest IQs at age 8 or 9. The lowest IQ children were among the least resilient.

4. **A high IQ equates to a healthier and longer life:** Ian Deary, a researcher at the University of Edinburgh, has been studying a group of 80-year-olds for whom he has childhood IQ records. The high scorers, he found, are the most successful in terms of health, longevity, and daily functioning.

    Similarly, researchers in the field of cognitive epidemiology find that people with lower IQs are less healthy and die younger. For example, in 2001, Whalley and Deary published a paper in the *British Medical Journal* in which they stated that **a drop of 15 points in IQ translates to a 24% increase in morbidity and a 21% lower chance of living beyond age 76.**

5. **You may need proof of giftedness:** If your child is gifted, an early IQ test may confirm the need for a special curriculum at kindergarten or school. To convince educators that your child is above average intelligence and may need special attention, evidence in the form of the results from a recognised IQ test will most likely be required.

6. **It helps identify any weaknesses in other areas:** Your child's intellectual ability may be obvious, but abilities in other areas such as muscle coordination and perceptual skills are less easily identifiable through observation alone. IQ testing may reveal any weakness of this nature and will enable you and educators

to assist children in overcoming these weaknesses or at least minimising the impact of them.

7. **It gives you a baseline to track progress:** Test scores provide baseline information for continued monitoring of a child's intellectual growth and progress. Early testing gives you the information you need to take any action you deem necessary sooner rather than later.

NOTE: Test score results may not meet your expectations – they may not be as high as you expected or hoped for. If this is the case, you may be inclined to lose confidence in your child. **Please do not do this.** Instead, use the information to apply some of the techniques listed in the book and to make informed decisions about your child's future.

INTRODUCTION

"Our greatest national resource is the minds of our children."

Walt Disney, American film producer

Intelligence has always been highly valued. To be labelled as being of "below average intelligence" can be a curse in more ways than one. Every parent wants their child to be intelligent and successful. Increasing a child's IQ is one of the stepping stones to giving that child the confidence and intellectual capability to perform well in a highly competitive world.

As a 2011 article in www.sciencemag.com pointed out, "Kids who score higher on IQ tests will, on average, go on to do better in conventional measures of success in life: academic achievement, economic success, even greater health, and longevity." Although IQ is not the entirety of intelligence, it is one of the key measures of intelligence. Science has shown that by helping your child increase their IQ, you can help them increase their intelligence and greatly benefit them in other areas of life.

Having worked in multiple, fast-moving corporate environments for the past 30 years, I have noticed how, in general, people with certain qualities quickly get noticed and often end up on the fast track. To succeed in these environments, qualities such as the ability to proactively research, absorb, and then apply knowledge have become the norm. Similarly, the ability to perceive and quickly analyse patterns is vital for jobs such as working on a trading desk in an investment bank. Even more challenging is the fact that often, there is a need to work fast whilst maintaining focused attention under pressure. These abilities among others are the ones that are evaluated during IQ tests.

I have always been interested in learning. In fact, books, education, and music have been an integral part of my life for as long as I can remember. My father continually stressed the importance of education. He was an extraordinarily intelligent man who, after my grandfather died, started work at the age of 11 in rural India. Despite the hard life that he endured, he became fluent in six languages, mastered classical music, and was a master craftsman. He was dedicated to learning and had cupboards full of books. He died when I was thirteen, but not before he had implanted in me a desire to constantly learn. He was a magnificent role model and both he and my brother inspired me to take advantage of all the educational opportunities available to me.

With my education, I was armed to enter and succeed in the corporate arena. Along the way, my two daughters and my son came into my life. As they grew and I continued to gain a better understanding of how the mind works, my interest in how the mind can be trained and tuned intensified. I witnessed how my children's thoughts and external events shaped their reality. It struck me that, with the right information, any parent can tweak a child's thinking and environment to help them to excel - not only academically but in all aspects of life. Over time, I committed to creating a set of guidelines that my children and other parents could use to help realise their own children's potential. This book is the first of these guidelines.

Many of the environmental, nutritional, health, and other challenges that we all face in the world today can have a direct impact on perceived intelligence. Any effect that we see in adults is often magnified in children. This book brings together several science-backed techniques to increase a child's IQ and decrease the impact of those factors that may reduce IQ.

Although the book is aimed at children's IQs, much of the information also applies to adults. Caregivers play a very important role in nurturing intelligence and the many other attributes required for success. If parents strive for better themselves, then children often follow suit. If you are a parent, undertake this journey jointly with your children and you will all benefit not only with a higher IQ, but with better health.

Most of the information is based on heavily-researched science-backed concepts, but some novel approaches are also presented. The information is valuable and deserves to be widely shared.

The children of today are the future of the world and it is our duty to ensure that we do our utmost to help these future generations achieve their true potential.

SECTION 1

PRECONCEPTION, PREGNANCY, AND PARENTS

1

Age, Diet, and Genetics of Parents before Conception

"Intelligence emerges from the interaction of a person's genetic makeup and the environment in which they develop. We have little control over nature's contribution, but the uterine environment is of critical importance and often overlooked by new parents."

Thomas J. Darvill, PhD, Chairman of Psychology, Oswego State University, New York

IQ has been shown — to a degree — to be inherited, and researchers have discovered that the "quality" of the parents' genome can be impacted by several factors including age and diet. In this chapter, we'll look at some of these factors, how they impact parents, and the potential consequences on the IQ of a child once it has been conceived.

Every part of our body, including the brain and the nervous system, is built according to instructions encoded in the genes that have been handed down from our parents. It seems reasonable, therefore, to assume that the intelligence of a child will, to a greater or lesser extent mirror the intelligence of its parents. This is in fact what researchers have discovered — the children of parents with high IQs tend to have high IQs whilst children of parents with low IQs tend to have low IQs.

In a recent study (2014) published in *Molecular Psychiatry*, Dr Beben Benyamin and his team from the University of Queensland analysed genetic data and IQ scores from 18,000 children aged 6 to 18 from Australia, the Netherlands, the UK, and the U.S. The analysis established that up to 40% of a child's intelligence is passed down from their parents.

Similarly, scientists from the Medical Research Council Social and

Public Health Sciences Unit in Glasgow interviewed 12,686 young people between the ages of 14 and 22 every year from 1994. They found the best predictor of intelligence was the IQ of the mother.

But it's not only IQ that's inherited. In a 2009 paper published in *Psychological Science*, geneticists Corina Greven and Robert Plomin studied the heritability of self-confidence and its relationship to IQ and performance. They concluded that self-confidence is not just a state of mind, but *a genetic trait*. From studying more than 3,700 pairs of twins aged between seven and ten, they found that children's self-confidence is greatly influenced by heredity – at least to the same degree that IQ is. Furthermore, these self-confidence genes seem to influence a child's school performance independently of IQ genes.

Robert Plomin identified that specific genes predict high intelligence, reading disability, and mental retardation. He found that the degree to which genetics accounts for differences in IQ varies from about 40% in pre-school years to about 80% in adulthood.

How the mother's diet before pregnancy affects the child's intelligence

The neural tube in an embryo is the precursor to the central nervous system. A 2011 paper published in the *Food Nutrition* bulletin looked at the effects of folate and vitamin B12 deficiency on brain development in children. Folic acid is the synthetically produced version of folate. The researchers found that a deficiency in folic acid prior to conception and in the early days of pregnancy (the periconceptional period) contributes to defects in the hollow structure from which the brain and spinal cord form – the neural tube.

In the same paper, the researchers found that vitamin B12 deficiencies have negative consequences on brain development during infancy and that deficits of both folic acid and vitamin B12 are linked to a greater risk of depression during adulthood.

According to Cochrane (an independent network of health researchers - www.cohcrane.org), folic acid supplementation is recommended for women **from the point that they are trying to conceive to the 12th week of pregnancy**.

The World Health Organization (WHO) recommends intermittent (weekly) iron and folic acid supplementation for all women of reproductive age, especially in populations where anaemia is commonly above 20%.

Diet before conception affects both fertility and the development of the baby, especially during the very early stages of pregnancy.

Does your diet affect your genes?

Genes are made of a chemical called DNA, which is short for deoxyribonucleic acid. Although we have no control over the genes that are handed down to us by our parents, we do have a degree of control over how our genes function. The food that we eat has been shown to influence how genes function. What you eat directly determines the genetic messages your body receives. This is the new science of nutrigenomics.

Research published in *The FASEB Journal* (September 2012) reported that the diet of mothers before they become pregnant chemically alters their DNA. This change in DNA in turn alters the DNA of their children.

But it's not only the diet of mothers that is an influencing factor in the DNA of children. A Boston University researcher, Dr Gladys Friedler, who has spent more than 40 years studying how the health of a father affects his children, states: *"It takes two to tango. Males are as important as females in terms of their impact on the foetus and in later development."*

Men who drink and smoke could be putting the health of their future children and grandchildren at risk. Toxic chemicals in cigarettes and alcohol are believed to lead to changes in the DNA. This modified DNA is then passed on to future generations via sperm. Stephen J. Schoenthaler, PhD, a professor of nutrition and behaviour at California State University in Long Beach, recommends that even before conception, the mother and probably the father should avoid tobacco, drugs and alcohol. Caffeine should also be limited.

Drugs, alcohol, and tobacco have long been known to impact health in a variety of ways but why, you may wonder, is there a restriction on caffeine? In 2006, Schmid et al reported that caffeine intake affected sperm DNA in healthy non-smokers (average age 46.4 years). Their research, which was published in *Human Reproduction*, concluded that men who drink more than 3 cups of coffee per day have increased sperm DNA damage. This damage may take the form of abnormal chromosomes, which may lead to gene mutations after fertilisation. These, in turn, increase the risks of developmental problems and genetic diseases among children.

> *It is not enough to clean up your diet during pregnancy. If you want to transmit healthy genes to a child, both men and women must adopt good dietary habits well before pregnancy.*

What is the ideal age to conceive?

Nowadays, both men and women are waiting longer to have children. They want to become established in their life and career. But is this a wise strategy to produce children of above average intelligence?

A recent Australian study lead by Dr John McGrath, a psychiatrist and epidemiologist at the Queensland Brain Institute in Brisbane, Australia, unearthed a surprising connection between the age of parents and the IQ of their offspring.

He reported that children born to older mothers with younger fathers have a better chance of having a higher IQ than children born to fathers who are older.

Dr McGrath's finding was supported by another study that tested the IQ of more than 33,000 U.S. children at the ages of 8 months, 4 years and 7 years. The results of this study demonstrated that children of whose fathers were older than the mother scored lower on intelligence tests than children whose mothers were older than the father. Both studies indicate that pairing an older mother with a younger father might produce children with higher IQs.

Nature (August 2012) recently reported that as men age, the amount of genetic damage transported in sperm increases, and therefore, the chance of a child having autism or some other defect at birth increases. The researchers discovered that, at the age of 20, a man transmits around 25 genetic mutations. This number increases to an average of 65 by the age of 40. Women, on the other hand, transmit about 15 genetic mutations, whatever their age.

Researchers at the Karolinska Institute in Sweden and Indiana University analysed data on more than two million children born between 1973 and 2001. They compared the data from children born to men aged 45 to those born to men aged 24. They found that children of older men were more likely to have a lower IQ. In addition, children of older men were 13 times more likely to have ADHD, 3.5 times more likely to have autism, and 25 times more likely to have bipolar disorder.

Men are susceptible to many more genetic mutations than women as they age. Therefore, the ideal man/woman combination to produce smart children is one in which the man is younger than the woman. A point to bear in mind, however, is that beyond the forties, risks associated with later pregnancy increase.

To measure the effect of a mother's age on their child, researchers from the London School of Economics examined data from the Millennium Cohort Study, which monitors the development of 18,000 children in the UK. They determined that children who are born to women in their thirties achieved the best cognitive scores. These children surpassed children born to women in their twenties and women in their forties.

In terms of a child's IQ, the best age for a mother-to-be to become pregnant is in her thirties. A woman who has a child in her thirties with a younger man increases the chances of their children having a higher IQ.

Other genetic dangers that should be considered

Cousin (consanguineous) marriages: Even though they are a well-known risk factor for genetic disorders that lead to intellectual and developmental disabilities, cousin marriages are widely practiced in many cultures. In 2016, a study of 221 children, of which 136 were from consanguineous marriages, was published in the journal *Frontiers in Public Health*. Almost 70% of the consanguineous children had a moderate intellectual disability, around 20% had severe intellectual disability, and 10% had another developmental disorder.

In Jordan (Hamamy et al, 2007), 20–30% of all marriages are between cousins. Of these, 69% are first cousins. Among families of first cousin marriages, around 30% had the highest rate of genetic disorder conditions such as intellectual disability.

In Qatar (16), of 1,515 women studied, 54% were in consanguineous marriages and the most common form was again between first cousins. The children of these women had a significantly higher rate of intellectual disability, asthma, diabetes, and epilepsy compared with children of non-consanguineous couples.

Sickle cell anaemia (SCA): SCA is an inherited blood disorder. If you are a carrier, you can pass these conditions on to your baby. *The Journal of the American Medical Association* published a paper titled *Neuropsychological Dysfunction and Neuroimaging Abnormalities in Neurologically Intact Adults with Sickle Cell Anaemia* (2001). The researchers compared the IQ of people with SCA against a control group and found that patients with SCA had an IQ 8.5 points lower.

SCA can be carried by anyone immaterial of race. However, it is more common among people of African, Caribbean, Mediterranean, Indian, Pakistani, South and Southeast Asian, and Middle East heritage.

Prospective parents and pregnant women from these backgrounds should have a blood test to see whether they are carriers of SCA. If you are a carrier, you need to discuss the matter with your licenced health practitioner to assess your options.

THINGS TO CONSIDER BEFORE CONCEIVING

Even before they conceive, prospective parents can take many steps to maximise the IQ of their future children:

- Work on yourself to become more intelligent and this will be passed down to your children to some degree. By doing this, not only will you pass on better genes to your child, but you will also be a powerful role model after they are born.

- If you want intelligent children, find an intelligent partner. Someone who is at least as intelligent as you, or more intelligent than you.

- Cut down or eliminate drugs, alcohol, tobacco, and caffeine to keep your DNA and sperm in pristine condition — even to the extent of avoiding indirect influences such as secondary smoke.

- If you're a woman, the best age to conceive is in your thirties. If your partner is younger than you, then this can work in your favour.

- If you're a man, the best age to conceive is when your partner is between 30-40 years of age. If you are older than her, then take extra care to stay healthy. Be aware though, that later pregnancies can have greater risks associated with them – both for mother and child.

- If your culture allows it, avoid cousin marriages.

2

The Mother's Diet, Nutrition, and Other Factors During Pregnancy

"The more we learn about the role of early nutrition in later cognition function, the more important it becomes to ensure that every child is adequately nourished during this sensitive period of brain development."

Lise Eliot, Professor of Neuroscience

Although the early years of life are critical to brain development, brain health actually starts in the womb. It is significantly affected by the mother's health prior to and during pregnancy. The mother's mental state, diet, nutrition, and overall fitness during and even before pregnancy are all aspects that influence the development of a baby in the womb. In this chapter, we'll examine the importance of some of these factors and the impact they can have on the IQ of a child after birth.

Nutritional influences during pregnancy

First let's consider some nutritional influences relevant to IQ:

Protein – Protein is a key nutrient in building the brain of a baby as well ensuring that the mother stays healthy throughout pregnancy.

Folate and Vitamin B12 – As described in the previous chapter, folate and vitamin B12 contribute to neural tube development and brain development in the baby.

Vitamin D – There are two types of vitamin D, vitamin D_2 and vitamin D_3. Research by Heaney et al published in 2011 established that vitamin D_3 is up to 87% more potent than vitamin D_2 in raising blood levels of vitamin D. Also, to become the active form, both vitamin D_2 and vitamin D_3 must undergo conversion within the body. Vitamin D_3 is converted 500% faster than vitamin D_2.

Dr Eva Morales and colleagues from the Center for Research in Environmental Epidemiology in Spain measured the vitamin D_3 levels in 1820 pregnant women. When they were 14 months of age, the children of these women were subject to neurocognitive and psychomotor testing. The results, as published in *Pediatrics* (2012), concluded that the children of mothers with vitamin D_3 levels above 30 ng/ml during pregnancy, had mental and psychomotor scores that were 3.17 and 2.42 higher, respectively, than children of mothers with vitamin D_3 levels lower than 20 ng/ml.

Sunshine is the best source of vitamin D. Other sources include cheese, beef liver and fatty fish such as tuna, mackerel and salmon. Many foods such as cereals are fortified with vitamin D. Vitamin D supplements are also readily available.

Iodine – Iodine is essential to the development of a baby's brain and nervous system. It regulates the rate at which the body uses energy (metabolism) and plays an important role in regulating the mother's thyroid gland. A deficiency of iodine, particularly in the first 12 weeks, is linked to significantly lower IQ in children.

In a study published in 2013, scientists from the universities of Surrey and Bristol found that during their pregnancy, 67% of 100 mothers who were studied had levels of iodine below the level recommended by the World Health Organization. When the children of these mothers were at the age of eight, they scored 3 points lower on verbal IQ compared to children born to mothers with adequate iodine. At age nine, they also had poorer reading ability.

Studies conducted in China found that extreme Iodine deficiency resulted in children with an IQ of 12.45 points lower than the average. Once iodine supplementation was introduced, the IQ increased so significantly that, 3.5 years later, the IQ gap had lessened to only 3.75 points.

The following foods are rich in iodine and should form a part of an expectant mother's diet: kelp, cranberries, organic yoghurt, organic strawberries, potatoes, and cheese. If necessary, iodine supplements could be taken.

Choline – Choline is an important nutrient that helps a baby's brain and spinal cord develop properly. Dr Gerald Weissmann, editor-in-chief of the *Federation of American Societies for Experimental Biology (FASEB) Journal*, stated that adequate choline during pregnancy boosts the intelligence of the unborn baby. Choline is vital to the development of those parts of a baby's brain that are linked to memory and recall.

Boeke and a team of researchers published a paper in the *American Journal of Epidemiology* (2013) that reported a higher choline intake during weeks 13 to 27 of pregnancy resulted in children with slightly better child visual memory at age 7.

Although not applicable to pregnant mothers, choline intake has been strongly linked to prostate cancer. For this reason, expectant mothers should consult with a certified nutritionist or doctor to ensure that they are taking appropriate levels of choline.

Choline rich foods include: cruciferous vegetables, peanuts, dairy products, eggs, meat, poultry and fish. Again, there are supplements available if the need arises

Omega-3 – Omega-3 oils provide many of the acids that a baby's brain needs during the growth spurt after week 28 of pregnancy and in the first months of life after birth. Researchers lead by Ingrid Helland gave pregnant and breastfeeding women daily cod liver oil tablets. They discovered that children born to mothers who had taken cod liver oil tablets during pregnancy and lactation had higher mental processing scores at 4 years of age compared with children of mothers who had taken corn oil.

Omega 3 fatty acids can be obtained from flaxseed oil, chia seeds, fatty fish, seafood, soybeans, walnuts, fish roe (eggs) and spinach.

Fruit — Increased fruit consumption during pregnancy results in infants that have higher cognitive performance. Canadian researchers from the University of Alberta looked at data from nearly 700 Edmonton children. They found that by the age of 1, the infants of pregnant women who ate six to seven servings of fruit a day, scored 6 – 7 points higher on IQ.

Despite the positive effects on IQ, senior study author Dr. Piush Mandhane cautioned against overconsumption of fruit during pregnancy due to the naturally high sugar content. If a decision is made to consume more fruit, ensure that the additional sugar from the fruit is counter-balanced by reducing the amount of sugar consumed through other means.

Poor nutrition and nutritional deficiencies lead to children with a lower than average IQ.

Other influencers during pregnancy

Apart from nutrition, the following factors during pregnancy have all been shown to influence the IQ of a child.

Alcohol has long been discouraged during pregnancy. Recent research suggests the effect of alcohol depends on whether the mother has a gene variant that affects how her body processes alcohol. Mothers with the variant who drank between 1 and 6 units a week during pregnancy had children with **lower IQ scores at age 8. The child's IQ was on average 2 points lower** for each genetic variant they had.

Tobacco use during pregnancy has been consistently associated with lower IQ throughout childhood. In a series of follow-ups conducted in the Ottawa Prenatal Prospective Study (OPPS) study, the children of women who ingested 16mg nicotine through smoking tobacco during pregnancy had a mean IQ **8 points lower** than those of unexposed children.

Medication is another factor that must be considered during pregnancy. As an example, *The Lancet Neurology* published research in 2013 indicating that the anti-epileptic drug, valproate affects the IQ of children when taken during pregnancy. The results revealed that children of mothers who had used valproate during pregnancy had IQ scores 7-10 points lower than children of mothers who had taken other antiepileptic drugs that were included in the study.

If you are taking medication before or during pregnancy, talk with your doctor about any concerns you may have about the medication affecting the intellectual health of your child. Ask if they know of any negative effects associated with the prescribed medicine. Beyond this, be proactive and do some research yourself. Either way, you should never self-medicate or come off your medication without first consulting your doctor.

Weight gain is something that is expected during pregnancy. However, gaining too much weight can lead to problems. It may lead to a large baby, which may result in a difficult delivery. This can be risky for the baby's brain. On the other hand, not gaining enough weight has been linked to a lower IQ because the baby will tend to have a smaller head and brain. The ideal weight gain, according to obstetricians, is between 25 to 35 pounds.

Alcohol consumption, tobacco use, medication, and excess or insufficient weight gain during pregnancy can all negatively impact the IQ of a child.

Exercise during pregnancy can be a good thing for a child's IQ. A study presented at The American Physiological Society stated that exercise may improve foetal breathing movements and autonomous nervous system development. Similarly, researchers at the University of Montreal found that as little as 20 minutes of exercise three times per week during pregnancy can increase a new-born's brain activity.

Aerobic exercise increases mitochondrial activity in a mother's brain and this increase crosses the placenta to benefit the foetal brain as well.

Richard E. Nisbett, author of *Intelligence and How to Get It*, says that "Children whose mother exercised 30 minutes a day score around **8 points higher on standard IQ tests** than children whose mothers were more sedentary."

Studies show that mothers who continue to work out during pregnancy have smarter babies.

Late-term birth also influences the IQ of children. A report in *JAMA Pediatrics* (2016) stated that late-term infants (born in the 41st week of pregnancy) have higher standardized test scores when they reach school-age compared with full-term (39 or 40 week) gestation. A greater percentage were classified as gifted.

The British Medical Journal published a study in 2003 led by Annette Wind Olsesen that examined the risk of recurring prolonged pregnancies. The researchers found that women whose first pregnancy lasted for 41 weeks instead of the normal 40 weeks had a 20% chance that the second pregnancy would also be prolonged. If the first pregnancy lasted for 44 weeks, the risk increased to 30%. Interestingly, however, if the woman had changed partners between pregnancies, the risk of a second prolonged pregnancy was reduced to 15%. This led researchers to believe that birth timing may be affected by the father's genes!

Stress is a contributing factor in many human health conditions and pregnancy is no exception. Numerous studies have shown that high levels of stress during pregnancy harms children. One of these studies, published in January 2007, investigated the intelligence of more than 100 babies and toddlers whose mothers had experienced extraordinarily high levels of stress in pregnancy. Professor Vivette Glover reported that the IQ of these children was generally several points below average. In addition to a low IQ, many of these children had higher than average levels of anxiety and attention deficit problems.

Stress is harmful to the IQ of your unborn child. Reduce stress by any means possible. Many people have used methods such as yoga, meditation, mindfulness, listening to calming music, visualisation, breathing exercises, and walking in nature to calm themselves.

THINGS TO DO DURING PREGNANCY

The mother's age, diet, genetics, and overall health all have a direct impact on the IQ of a child. To reduce any risks associated with these factors, mothers-to-be need to:

- Make sure that the mother's body has the right levels of vitamins, minerals and micro-nutrients. Work with your GP, the pre-natal clinic, and a qualified nutritionist to determine whether you need to address any deficiencies.

- Avoid alcohol, tobacco, and secondary smoke.

- Avoid any unnecessary stress or trauma. If you suffer from anxiety, consider taking up a mind calming practice such as yoga or meditation.

- If you are on medication, check that it does not have any undesirable effects on the baby – do your own research and discuss the findings with your doctor. Do not self-medicate – always consult a doctor.

- Make sure your weight is in the appropriate range for your body type.

- Exercise for at least 20 minutes a day every day.

3

Breastfeeding and IQ

"While breastfeeding may not seem the right choice for every parent, it is the best choice for every baby."

- Amy Spangler, author, breastfeeding expert, and president of baby gooroo

Breastfeeding a baby is widely advocated as having many benefits such as protection from infectious diseases and a reduction in mortality. The link between breastfeeding and IQ is hotly debated, but there are more studies supporting the breastfeeding IQ link than there are denouncing it.

Evidence supporting the positive effect of breastfeeding on IQ

A study by Cesar G Victora and colleagues published in *The Lancet Global Health* in 2015 examined the association between breastfeeding and intelligence, educational attainment, and income. It was launched in 1982 and followed 5,914 Brazilian babies from all backgrounds. Between 2012 and 2013, the researchers were able to obtain data about IQ and breastfeeding duration of 3,493 of the original participants.

The analysis showed that children who were breastfed for 12 months or more had an IQ score that was 3.76 points higher. On average, they also had 0.91 more years of education and higher monthly incomes than children who were breastfed for less than 1 month. The researchers concluded that breastfeeding does increase IQ and that IQ was responsible for 72% of the effect on income.

The Journal of the American Medical Association published an article in May 2008 titled *Breastfeeding and Child Cognitive Development*. The research is based on the long-term follow-up of 17,046 mothers and children who were part of a research project in the Republic of Belarus. In the article, researchers reported an increase of up to 7.5 IQ points in elementary age children who were breastfed, as well as an increase in verbal performance.

Despite the evidence, there is a debate surrounding the value of breastfeeding in relation to IQ. Critics argue that other factors associated with a mother's choice to breastfeed e.g. higher socioeconomic status, level of education, and different child-rearing attitudes might promote cognitive development more than the actual act of breastfeeding. However, several studies — including work by Kramer et al, *Breastfeeding and Child Cognitive Development* (May 2008) and Anderson et al, *Breast-feeding and cognitive development: a meta-analysis* (October 1999) — concluded that even after appropriate adjustments, breastfeeding was associated with an advantage of around 3 points on tests of cognition in children born at term and around 5 points in those born pre-term.

An early study conducted in the late 1980s compared the IQ scores of 345 Scandinavian children at age 5. The children who were breastfed for less than three months had an IQ score that was 7 points lower than the children who were breastfed for six months.

Evidence denouncing the IQ increasing benefits of breastfeeding

Against the background of research supporting the IQ-increasing benefits of breastfeeding, it is worth mentioning one recent piece of research that found no link between breastfeeding and IQ. Dr Sophie Von Stumm used data involving more than 15,000 families and derived from the *Twins Early Development Study (TEDS)*. The twins' intelligence was assessed at 2, 3, 4, 7, 9, 10, 12, 14, and 16 years. The results, published in *PLOS ONE* (September 2015), concluded that breastfeeding has little benefit for early life intelligence and cognitive growth from toddlerhood through adolescence.

Does the timing of feeds influence IQ?

A recent study published in the *European Journal of Health* (March 2012 edition) found that the academic performance of breast-fed or bottle-fed babies who are fed to a schedule is inferior to their demand-fed peers. The researchers, from the University of Essex and the University of Oxford, based their findings on the results of IQ tests and school SATs tests of children between the ages of 5 and 14. The results showed that the IQs of 8 year olds who were demand-fed were between 4 and 5 five points higher than the scores of schedule-fed children. This difference, between schedule-fed and demand-fed children, is found regardless of whether the children are breastfed or bottle-fed babies.

So why do demand-fed babies fare better? Gwen Dewar PhD, in her 2017 online article *Jettisoning the infant feeding schedule: Why babies are better off feeding on cue* cites several reasons:

- A one size-fits-all feeding schedule may not be the best choice for your baby because different babies have different needs.

- Additionally, a mother's milk can fluctuate in quality from day to day and even during the day. Therefore, a schedule that worked yesterday may leave baby hungry today. Feeding a baby on-demand will help to make good any shortfalls due to fluctuations in the quality of milk.

- If new-borns are not fed when they show signs of being hungry — usually before they start to cry — there is a bigger risk of dehydration and underfeeding

- Frequent feeds help breastfeeding mothers establish a good milk supply.

What if breastfeeding is not fulfilling the nutritional needs of an infant?

Some mothers may feel that breast milk is not sufficient for their child. In these cases, the first thing to do is take advice from a midwife or doctor. It may be that there is no real issue if the baby is continuing to thrive. On the other hand, the doctor or midwife may advise supplementing breast milk with formula milk or some other course of action.

Whatever the case, the mother must ensure that **her** nutritional intake is adequate. In some regions of India, during the first weeks of nursing, the new mother is encouraged to eat a small bowl of specially blended "cereal" called Panjeeri. Panjeeri is made up of a number of ingredients including most of the following:

> Fennel seeds, turmeric, gum arabic, almonds, cashews, pistachios, ginger powder, ground cumin seeds, ground cardamom seeds, ghee, pumpkin/melon seeds, unrefined sugar, whole wheat flour, coconut oil, ground ajova seeds, lotus seeds, flame of the forest, and dried coconut.

Together, these ingredients form a very dense and nutritious meal, which works to promote a rich and full milk supply for baby and at the same time, support the recovery of the mother.

BREASTFEEDING IS GOOD FOR BABY'S IQ

The precise cause of higher IQs in breastfed babies is still being debated. It could be due to the nutritional makeup of breast milk or the extra physical contact between a mother and her child. Regardless, most studies indicate that breastfeeding has a positive effect on a child's IQ.

- It is advantageous for babies to be breastfed for as many months as is feasible. For example, three months is better than one month, six months is better than three months, and so on.

- Breastfeeding is beneficial for your child not only because it has been shown to possibly enhance IQ, but because breast milk contains antibodies that help your baby fight off viruses and bacteria.

- Feeding your baby on demand rather than on a schedule may lead to a 4-5 point IQ increase. This may require changes in your schedule, but if it helps your baby, then it's a small price to pay.

- Sometimes mothers who cannot or do not want to nurse their child feel a societal or family pressure to breastfeed. This can lead to internal conflict and stress which will probably outweigh any benefits that baby may derive from breastfeeding. In such cases, it's probably better to default to a good quality formula milk.

4

Parents

"Parents are the ultimate role models for children. Every word, movement, and action has an effect. No other person or outside force has a greater influence on a child than the parent."

Bob Keeshan, TV producer and actor

The role of parents and other significant adults has time and time again been demonstrated as a key factor in the success — academic or otherwise — of a child. Children whose parents are actively involved in the nurturing of their children daily have higher test scores, higher grades, better school attendance, greater motivation, and lower use of drugs and alcohol. In this chapter, we'll look at how parents and teachers influence a child's performance and IQ.

A study titled *The Effective Provision of Pre-School Education (EPPE) Project: Findings from the Pre-school Period* (2004) tracked the progress of more than 3,000 children in the UK since they were 3 years old. In the paper, the researchers state that *"what parents and carers do makes a real difference to young children's development...there are a range of activities that parents undertake with pre-school children which have a positive effect on their development … what parents do with their children is more important than who parents are. "*

They presented examples of activities parents can do with children that were all associated with higher intellectual and social/behavioural scores. These included: reading, teaching songs, painting and drawing, playing with letters and numbers, going on trips to the library and other places of interest, and play sessions at home with their friends.

The researchers asserted that *"Poor mothers with few qualifications can improve their children's progress and give them a better start at school by engaging in activities at home that engage and stretch the child's mind."*

> *In the book "50 Interviews: What it Takes to Make More Money Than Your Parents", 50 young entrepreneurs were interviewed about their journey to success. Many questions were asked, one of which was "What is your single most important reason for success?" In almost all cases, the answer was along the lines of "having supportive parents" or "having a supportive family."*

Being genuinely interested

Diana Divecha PhD is a developmental psychologist and research affiliate with the Yale Centre for Emotional Intelligence. She has guided parent education in the San Francisco Bay Area and currently writes about research on children's development and advises on matters relating to children and families.

On her blog (www.developmentalscience.com), she makes the point that when adults have a genuine interest in a child and enjoy their company, a rich interaction that teaches children on multiple levels is the outcome. Under these conditions of undivided attention and closeness, a child feels a sense of security, which helps to focus the child's learning.

She goes on to state that exposure to books, puzzles, and engaging verbal interactions was found to increase young children's IQs by more than 7 points.

> *Create a supportive, stimulating, and cognitively rich environment for your children. Have books lying around, word/phrase walls, graphics, pictures, and other mentally stimulating items. Repeated exposure to and interactions with multiple print and visual sources will help to boost their IQ.*

Security and support

One of the main jobs of parents is to provide security and reassurance for their children. In 1999, Crandell and Hobson studied 36 middle-class mothers and their 3 year olds. They found that children who felt psychologically secure, felt protected by their caregivers, and knew that they could depend on them scored 12 points higher than the children who felt insecure.

This finding was reinforced by a 2012 Washington University study published in the *Proceedings of the National Academy of Sciences* that demonstrated having a mother who is loving and nurturing significantly contributed to a child's eventual intelligence.

As adults, we acknowledge the importance of feeling safe and supported. One can only assume that whatever importance we, as adults, assigned to these feelings is magnified in children because they are dependent on caregivers.

> *Help your children to feel more secure through nurturing, hugs, and affection, verbal encouragement, daily routines, and assurance that you are there for them. Help them express their fears and worries to you.*

Talking with and listening to your child

Through various analyses, it's been known for many years that when adults speak with younger children, it encourages cognitive development. These studies show that encouraging a child to talk about and recall past events or describe experiences is particularly beneficial for cognitive development. In one study, the mothers of 20-month-old children were instructed on how to use open-ended questions to draw out a child's stories, how to be a good listener and how to encourage a child to pursue their interests. The children of mothers who applied this training demonstrated a 6 point increase in IQ.

Betty Hart and Todd Risley conducted a landmark study in which they identified 42 families across three socioeconomic classes: welfare, working class, and professional. Each of these families had new-born children who were born on the same day. When the children were 7 months old, researchers visited each family for one hour a month over a two-and-a-half-year period. During each visit, researchers taped and transcribed all conversations and actions that took place in front of the child.

At the end of the study, using the data they had collected, the researchers projected that by the time they reached kindergarten, the children of the professional family would have heard 45 million words, the children of the working-class family 26 million words and the children of the family on welfare only 13 million words. They went on to say that academic success correlated to the number of words the children had heard.

Hart and Risley wrote in their book *Meaningful Differences in the Everyday Experience of Young American Children*, "With few exceptions, the more parents talked to their children, the faster the children's vocabularies were growing and the higher the children's I.Q. test scores at age 3 and later."

Talking with your children often is important, as is asking open-ended questions and listening to them attentively. Answer their questions honestly, calmly, and factually, but don't overwhelm them with too much information. Help them share their feelings and have fun discussing things that you have experienced together.

The importance of praise

It is important to praise children, but a lot of parents struggle with finding the right balance when it comes to praising their children. Can you praise a child too much? When should you praise them? Is the amount of praise important?

Experts say that understanding when and where to praise children is important, but praising them in the right way is more important. In a number of experiments involving American 5th graders, researchers Claudia Mueller and Carol Dweck discovered that the way children behaved depended on the kinds of praise they received.

Children who were complimented on their **intelligence** by being told that they were smart tended to avoid challenges. They preferred easy tasks so that their risk of failure and looking less intelligent was reduced. They tended to:

- Give up after a failure and view their failures as evidence of low intelligence

- Have worse performance after a failure
- Misrepresent how well they did on a task
- Be more interested in how they measured up relative to others rather than learning how to improve their future performance

On the other hand, children who were commended for their **effort** displayed the opposite trend. These children:

- Sought tasks that were challenging that would enhance their learning
- Were more interested in learning new strategies for success rather than finding out how other children had performed

So, praise your children, but don't always praise them by telling them that they are smart. By being told that they are smart, kids become labelled as "smart" or label themselves that way. This prompts them to gear their efforts towards ensuring that they do not lose the label. They become frightened of failure, because in their eyes, if you fail, you cannot be smart.

> *Praising children is a positive thing to do, but you should praise them in a certain way. Praise them for their effort more than their intelligence. For example, "Well done! Nine out of ten is a great result. All the effort that you put in has really paid off!" is better praise than "Well done! Nine out of ten is a great result — you are so smart!"*

Physical and verbal abuse of children

Punishing children through spanking and similar punishments lowers their IQ. Murray Straus, from the University of New Hampshire, found that corporal punishment leads to a lower IQ. Since 1969, Straus has been researching the effects of corporal punishment on children and he has found that the IQ score of children who were physically punished was up to a five-points lower than children who weren't. The more spanking that took place, the lower the IQ. Interestingly, when Straus extended his research to study 32 countries, he found that in countries where spanking is acceptable, the average IQ of the population that was sampled was lower than in countries where spanking was infrequent.

Of course, abuse can also be verbal and sexual. Most parents have probably shouted at their children at one time or another and then probably regretted it after the event. Although undesirable, the occasional angry or harsh word may not impact a child for life. However, frequent verbal abuse will have profound and long-lasting negative effects.

In Amie Kolodziej's October 2015 online article (www.blog.allpsych. com), she lists several effects of child abuse. These include lower cognitive capacity, poorer language development, reduced academic achievement and lower IQ score. Similarly, IrigarayI et al (2013) cites dozens of references to studies that clearly show that maltreatment of children has a detrimental effect on reading scores, maths results, overall educational attainment and persistently low IQ.

So how does this link to verbal abuse? Teicher et al (2007) found that *"The effects of verbal abuse were worse than witnessing serious domestic violence and as serious as sexual abuse outside the home, but not as bad as sexual abuse by a family member"*. Based on this, we can assume that persistent verbal abuse, especially from parents has a negative impact on children

Spanking and other forms of physical and verbal abuse have a detrimental effect on a child's IQ. Not only that, the results may work in the short term but sustained physical punishments wreak havoc on the long-term development of children.

Socioeconomic Status (SES)

The Socioeconomic Status (SES) of an individual or group is their position within a social structure. SES depends on many things including education, occupation, income, accumulated wealth, and place of residence. Sophie von Stumm and Robert Plomin published the findings of a study that examined the role of SES on the IQ of children. The results were published in the journal *Intelligence* (2015) and indicated that on average, children from a lower SES environments perform more poorly on intelligence tests compared to children from higher SES environments. This difference is noted from the age of 2. By age 16, the difference in IQ between the two groups was **6 points.**

> *By working to better educate yourself, have a successful career, and increase your financial worth, you are not only securing a better lifestyle for yourself, but also increasing the probability of your children having a higher IQ.*

PARENTS ARE ROLE MODELS

Parents are a child's first role models and their attitudes towards their children are major contributors to the success and happiness of a child. Some of the many things you could do to help improve your child's IQ through your role as a caregiver include:

- If you want your children to succeed, you need to be actively involved with them every day. Spend time with them. Talk with them. Ask them open-ended questions. Be genuinely interested in them and enjoy them and their achievements.

- Improve your vocabulary, read more, keep on improving and learning. Always remember you are a role model for your child. As you continue to better yourself, it will have a positive effect on your children.

- Work to improve your SES by better educating yourself, increasing your income and financial standing, and, if possible, moving to a better neighbourhood with more spacious accommodation.

- Create an environment in which children can both learn and express themselves. Engage them in activities with books, puzzles, and interesting verbal interactions.

- Believe in your children and their potential — have a positive view of them. Be careful not to plant any limiting beliefs in their mind.

- Be liberal but sincere with your praise. Praise them more for the effort that they put in rather than their intelligence alone.

- At times, children may need to be disciplined. Rather than resorting to spanking, verbal abuse or other forms of punishment, find other, less traumatic ways to make your point.

5

Environmental and Social Influences

"To assist a child, we must provide him with an environment which will enable him to develop freely."

Maria Montessori, Italian educator and physician

The environment in which children live and work is of critical importance to their early learning and development. Where a child lives, the school, the degree and type of stimulation that they receive at home, the noise and the amount of space are all factors that contribute to and influence the development of that child. In this chapter, we look at several of these environmental factors and how they influence IQ.

The home environment

In 1989, the American Psychological Association published a study titled *Home Environment and Cognitive Development in the First 3 Years of Life*. The study revealed that facets of the child's environment at home, such the responsiveness of parents and the availability of stimulating play materials, were strongly related to a child's development — even more than the socioeconomic status (SES) of the parents.

A dramatic example of how much environment can impact IQ was demonstrated in what has come to be known as the *"1938 Glenwood Project"*. In this study, the researcher H. Skeels took two children from an orphanage and placed them on the adult women's ward in the state institution at Glenwood. When these children, who were originally classified as *"retarded"*, were moved to the women's ward, Skeels saw an *"astonishing"* increase in the IQ of the children.

After this success with two children, Skeels, moved all the children whose IQ tested as retarded to the state institution at Glenwood. All the children were 3 years old and had an initial mean IQ of 64.3. A control group that remained in the orphanage had a mean IQ of 86.7. After 18 months, the IQ of the children who had been moved increased by 27.5 points whilst the IQ of the control group decreased by 26.2 points.

This remarkable result can, at least in part, be attributed to the overwhelming attention and love that the children received from their new mothers. The children were given toys to play with, taken on trips and the substitute mothers were taught how to draw out language from the children and intellectually stimulate them.

The Glenwood Project clearly demonstrated that IQ can increase or decrease depending upon the environment. This is an extraordinary example, but it clearly illustrates the profound effect that environment can have on IQ.

The impact of crowding in the home

Personal space is a region of physical space that surrounds us and in which we feel safe and comfortable. If this personal space is breached it can make us feel uneasy. Working and living in a crowded environment can violate our personal space with the result that the way we behave and function is affected.

There is no standard definition for crowding. What is viewed as crowded in one culture is considered normal in another. Researchers too, define crowding differently. *Definitions of Crowding and the Effects of Crowding on Health: A Literature Review (2001)* presents the standards used by some regulatory bodies and researchers. By way of example, the British bedroom standard as listed in this document states that a separate bedroom is required for each of the following:

- a married couple
- any person aged 21 or over
- a pair of adolescents of the same sex aged 10-20
- a pair of children of the same sex under 10 years of age

JAGIR S. REEHAL, PH.D.

The British standard goes on to say that:

> *"Any unpaired person aged ten to 20 is paired, if possible, with a child under ten of the same sex. If that is not possible, that person is given a separate room as is an unpaired child under ten. Where the number of bedrooms is one or more below the bedroom standard, households are classified as overcrowded".*

Some of the research that has established that crowding has a negative impact on a child's development is presented below.

In a 2006 paper in the *Annual Review of Psychology*, Gary Evans reviewed how aspects of the physical environment affect a child's development. One of the factors he focused on was residential crowding. In the paper, he cited the work of several researchers who have found that residential crowding directly or indirectly affects the cognitive performance of children. The key findings were:

Age range	Effect noted
18-24 months	Negative correlation between crowding and mental development
30 months	IQ scores negatively impacted
30, 36 and 42 months	Negative impact on verbal, perceptual, and quantitative performance
Elementary school	Poorer performance on standardised reading tests with a resultant self-perception of being less competent at school
High school – age 25	Negative impact on school performance through high school and educational attainment at age 25

The results of a study similar to that of Evans' was published in the *International Journal of Psychology*, (2013). In this paper, the authors, Ferguson et al, cited several researchers who discovered that:

- In crowded homes, parents talk less to their children. When they did talk, these parents used vocabulary and sentence structures that were simpler than families who live in uncrowded homes.

- Children who came from crowded homes spent more of their time unoccupied and less time engaged in play with objects.
- Children's development of physical and quantitative skills suffered in crowded houses.
- Apartment square footage was inversely related to school performance.
- The negative associations between residential density and decreased academic achievement extended into secondary school.

Having a spacious environment in which to live and work aids a child's cognitive development. Crowded homes can be harmful not only to child's academic performance, but they may also lead to behavioural and health problems – effects that can last a lifetime. Ensure that you dedicate enough time for each child and that every child has enough room for them to complete activities such as homework, and to just sit and be in their own space.

Consequences of noisy environments

Homes are often filled with an assortment of noises from TVs to washing machines, driers, traffic, and even jets flying overhead. In 2008, Charlotte Clark published a paper summarizing the latest research into the influence of noise on performance and behaviour.

In her paper, she discusses an experiment in which it was found that noise affected verbal and non-verbal performance. Three groups of children were tested. Group one was the control group - they were tested in a quiet environment. Group two was tested in an environment where there was only ambient background noise. Group three was tested in an environment where there were children talking (babble) over the ambient background noise. The results showed that compared to group one, group two children performed most poorly on verbal literacy tasks whilst the performance of group three children was significantly poorer on non-verbal processing tasks.

Environmental influences on IQ and other cognitive functions can be dramatic. The impact of these influences is stronger in early childhood and can either increase or decrease the IQ of a child.

Domestic violence

Unfortunately, domestic violence is a global problem that is common in many households. Recent UK statistics indicate that on average, police receive a call about domestic abuse every 30 seconds. In the UK, domestic abuse cases now account for over 14% of all court prosecutions. Extreme stress and violence can be deeply traumatic for anyone. For children, domestic violence and stress can lead to trauma that negatively affects their personality, confidence and IQ.

In *Development and Psychopathology* (Spring 2003), Koenen et al published a paper in which they reported that extreme stress in childhood, such as domestic violence, affects children's neurocognitive development, which results in a lower IQ. Their study looked at a sample of 1,116 pairs of twins aged 5. The researchers asked mothers to report their experience of domestic violence over the past 5 years. It was found that pairs of twins exposed to high levels of domestic violence had, on average, an IQ that was 8 points lower than unexposed twins.

Stress and domestic violence can profoundly affect a child's IQ. Children who are exposed to such trauma become fearful and anxious. They are always on guard, watching and waiting for the next event to occur, and rarely feel safe. They are always worried for themselves, their mother, their siblings, and may feel worthless and powerless.

Bullying

Bullying is another common global problem that has now extended beyond face-to-face physical and verbal abuse to electronic bullying. In the U.S., up to 50% of children report being bullied at least once a month.

The effect of bullying can be so profound that as well as affecting a child's confidence and cognitive functioning, later in life, socioeconomic status (SES) and social life is also impacted. The damaging effects of bullying can persist for decades.

A British study published in the *American Journal of Psychiatry* (2014) measured the long-term effects of bullying on nearly 18,000 children in England, Scotland, and Wales born during one week in 1958. When the children were 7 and 11 years old, the parents of the children were contacted and interviewed about the degree of bullying their children had experienced. At the same time as the interviews, researchers measured the children's IQ score and examined teacher's reports for any behavioural problems that pointed to anxiety or depression. Then, at ages 23, 45, and 50, researchers checked in with roughly 8,000 of those children and noted their health, SES, and social wellbeing.

At the age of 50, the children who had been bullied — especially those who had been repeatedly bullied — lagged in educational attainment and memory tests. As a group, they had poorer cognitive function than people who were not bullied as children. They also reported increased anxiety, depression, suicidal thoughts, and poorer physical health.

How adoption can influence IQ

Adopting a child can be the only option for some people who want to be parents. For others, it is an opportunity to make a positive difference to the life a child who is not able to be with their birth parents.

In 1999, Capron and Duyme conducted a study to examine the influence of SES on adopted French children. The children were aged between four and six with initial IQs that averaged 77 – putting them close to retardation on the IQ scale. Most were neglected or abused in their early life, then moved from one institution or foster home to the next.

After 9 years, the children were re-tested, and every one of them performed better. The degree of improvement was directly linked to the socioeconomic status of the adopting family. *"Children adopted by farmers and laborers had average IQ scores of 85.5; those placed with middle-class families had average scores of 92. The average IQ scores of youngsters placed in well-to-do homes climbed more than 20 points, to 98."*

A study published in 2015 in the *Proceedings of the National Academy of Sciences* compared the cognitive ability of 436 sibling pairs in Sweden. One child was raised by biological parents whilst the other by adoptive parents. Between the ages of 18 and 20, the IQ of each sibling was measured and at the same time, each parent's education level was also rated on a five-point scale. Researchers found that the IQ of the children raised by their biological and typically less-educated parents was 4.4 points lower than siblings who had been adopted into higher-educated and more financially-secure families.

The researchers noted that previous studies had found that educated parents were more likely to talk at the dinner table, take their children to museums, and read stories to their children at night.

This paper supported an earlier paper that was published in the *Psychological Bulletin* (March 2005). The researchers Van Ijzendoorn, Juffer, and Poelhuis demonstrated that the IQ scores of adopted children – by moving to a different environment – were higher than their biological siblings who were not adopted. The analysis also showed that biologically-unrelated children raised together in the same home had some similarity in IQ scores.

Adoption, as well as affording a child a better life, can lead to an increase in IQ.

Social environments and feedback from others

As children, we all experienced the desire to fit into a social group at school. These groups may be based on ability such as being in the top set in Mathematics or being selected for the school football team. Once accepted into a group, certain criteria must continue to be met. But what happens if a group member fails to "perform" at the same level as others in the group?

Philosophical Transactions of the Royal Society B, (2012) published a study by a team of researchers from five institutions which examined how social influences affect mental abilities and decision-making skills. The research team created small groups with group members matched by their IQ. These groups were then assigned cognitive tasks against their peers within their groups. The results of the tasks were ranked and broadcast to everyone in the group during the course of the study.

Researchers discovered that this public broadcasting had a significant effect on the IQ of some participants – specifically those who had a low IQ to start with. The IQ of those who started with a low IQ dropped an average of 17.4 points during the study.

Lead author Kenneth Kishida noted that *"Our study highlights the unexpected and dramatic consequences even subtle social signals in group settings may have on individual cognitive functioning."*

Since most of a child's learning — both inside and outside the classroom — is in a social context, it is important, therefore, to understand that what children hear and see about their performance relative to their peers can drastically affect their performance.

ENVIRONMENT AFFECTS IQ

The environment has a clear effect on a child's development and IQ. Parents and caregivers should create an environment that is enriching and nurturing — an environment that encourages a child's growth in all areas. Here are some ideas to improve this:

- Have bookshelves in your house and populate them with books that are appropriate for your children.

- Make sure there are plenty of art and writing supplies around to allow encourage budding artists to express themselves freely.

- If you can, have a computer and or tablet PC that children can use, but ration its use and ensure that parental controls are activated.

- Be attuned and open enough to your children to be able to detect abnormal signs that could point to issues such as bullying. Children will often hide such issues from their parents.

- Work to make sure your child is resilient and able to bounce back from perceived negative feedback.

- Children need space. This may be difficult, but try to give children at least a small space where they can sit and work, write, paint, or draw.

- Where noise is concerned — keep it down as much as possible!

SECTION 2

EARLY YEARS
AND BEYOND

6

The Pre-school Advantage

"Experts tell us that 90% of all brain development occurs by the age of five. If we don't begin thinking about education in the early years, our children are at risk of falling behind by the time they start Kindergarten."

Robert. L. Ehrlich, American attorney and politician

Pre-school is beneficial for children in many ways, but before we explore this, we'll clarify what pre-school is, as it can be a confusing term. It is also known as nursery school, pre-primary school, or kindergarten outside the U.S. and UK. In some cases, pre-school refers to pre-kindergarten. In general, it is available to children between the ages of 2 and 5 although 3-5 is the more usual age range.

Pre-school is often a child's first experience in a structured setting — a foundation that will prepare children for the learning they will experience from elementary school onwards. As well as this, pre-school promotes social and emotional development, languages, cognitive skills, and a host of other benefits.

With respect to IQ, a study published in 2013 in *Perspectives on Psychological Science* carried out meta-analyses on the effect of pre-school on the IQ of over 7,000 young children. They found that:

- Attending pre-school can raise a child's IQ by more than 4 points.
- Children who attend pre-schools that contain a language development component can have an IQ boost of more than 7 points.

Children who attend pre-school have higher IQs because according to researchers, it offers novel stimuli, opportunities to practise problem-solving, and the chance to navigate social interactions — activities that may increase underlying intelligence. Because young children cannot define a world that they have not encountered, nor identify a picture of an item that they have never seen, pre-school may raise performance in intelligence tests merely by exposing young children to new information and vocabulary.

A study titled *The Effective Provision of Pre-School Education (EPPE) Project: Findings from the Pre-school Period* tracked the progress of more than 3,000 children in the UK since they were 3. The researchers published their findings in 2004 when the children were 7 years old after eliciting clear evidence. Here are some of the findings:

- Pre-school increases all-round development in children.
- An earlier start (under 3 years) is related to better intellectual development.
- Part-time attendance led to the same gains as full-time attendance.
- High-quality pre-schooling leads to enhanced intellectual and social/behavioural development in children. Indicators of high-quality include: a trained teacher as a manager for every child, an adequate number of trained teachers as staff, and warm, interactive relationships with other children.
- Children in pre-schools with staff that have better qualifications make more progress.
- Children make better all-round progress in pre-schools that view educational and social development as equally important and complementary.

Montessori pre-schools

The highest IQ gain during pre-school is to be found in **Montessori** pre-schools. Dr Maria Montessori was one of the most significant educators of the 20th century. Dr Montessori discovered that, during the early years, children learn best by doing. She noticed how happy and self-motivated learners create a positive image of themselves as confident and successful. Her aim was to develop the whole child through a holistic approach. To this end she produced specially-designed resources to encourage the development of independence and a love of learning from an early age.

In a study published in October 2015, Nooshin Ahmadpour and

Adis Kraskian Mujembari measured the impact of the Montessori teaching method on the IQ levels of a sample of 80 children aged 5 (40 children from the traditional kindergartens and 40 from a Montessori-regulated kindergarten) who were randomly selected from different kindergartens. Their results showed that children at the Montessori pre-school had an average IQ over 8 points higher than those at traditional pre-schools.

Pre-schooling at home

Some parents choose to pre-school at home. There may be many reasons for this — philosophical, financial, and religious. They may be unable to gain a place for their child in a pre-school of their choice. The parents may have been home educated themselves or may feel that the methods of teaching in school aren't right for their child and that they can provide a better education for their child at home.

Whatever the reasons, if parents can devote enough time and energy to their child's education, home pre-schooling is a viable option. Sylva et al (2004) found that in all cases of home-schooling, it is the quality of the learning environment at home that is most important for intellectual and social development. The parents' education, their occupation, or their income are less important. In other words, what parents do is more significant than who they are.

To make home schooling effective, include a variety of activities such as: teaching and playing with letters and numbers; reading interactively; teaching and playing songs and nursery rhymes; painting, drawing, and other creative activities; gardening; visits to the library and places of interest; and creating regular opportunities for them to play with their friends at home.

PRE-SCHOOL ENHANCES IQ

Young children are learning sponges. Every word they learn and every new experience is an investment in their future. Starting them on the path to formal learning sooner rather than later is something that will help them towards a higher IQ.

- Pre-school availability and funding varies from country to country and state to state. To find out what is available for your child, you should enquire with your local education authority.

- If you are interested, the Economist Intelligence Unit have prepared a report that ranks the pre-school environments in 45 countries. Just search online for "Starting Well Index".

- Montessori schools and other pre-schools can be found in most major towns in almost every country. Each school has its own admission procedure and fee structure. When looking for pre-schools, you may wish to consider the following:

  - Best option: Montessori pre-school
  - Second choice: Traditional pre-school with a language component
  - Third choice: Traditional pre-school without any language component

7

The Role of Teachers

"My teacher thought I was smarter than I was – so I was."

Anonymous 6-year-old

From the age of three until they leave school or college, teachers play a huge part in a child's life. In many cases, next to parents and family, teachers are often the biggest influence on a child. This influence can be so great that what a teacher knowingly or unknowingly believes or communicate about a child's abilities has been proven to affect how well that child performs.

In their book *Pygmalion in The Classroom*, Robert Rosenthal and Lenore Jacobson concluded that the intellectual development of students is affected by what teachers expect and how those expectations are communicated. They found that student performance and gains in IQ scores were significantly affected by teacher expectancies. In the research that lead to the book, Rosenthal found that students that teachers expected to succeed were given more approval, more time to answer, and more specific feedback. Also, teachers consistently acknowledged these children more through touching, nodding, and smiling.

More recently, in 2011 and 2014, Columbia and Harvard economists studied 20 years of data pertaining to 2.5 million students. They found that some teachers, categorised as value added (VA) teachers, who consistently succeeded in raising the standardized test scores of their students have a lasting influence on their students' lives. Their students are more likely to attend university, have a larger income, live in better neighbourhoods, and accumulate more savings for retirement. The research also discovered that whichever schools these VA teachers moved to, test scores increased. Likewise, when VA teachers left a school, test scores dropped.

Madon, Jussim, and Eccles (1997) demonstrated that teacher estimates of students' academic achievement potential had a role in predicting future achievement. From their observation of 1,539 children, they concluded that children whose potential is underestimated by parents or teachers may suffer low self-esteem and a cognitive performance that is less than they are capable of.

In her book, Child Development, Laura Berk states that if a child's parents and/or teachers develop a negative view of the child, the child will personally adopt that view of him or herself and perform accordingly.

Similarly, stereotyping is an issue that can seep into the psyche of children and remain there, unconsciously limiting their performance. American psychologist Sian Beilock conducted an experiment to demonstrate this, which was published in *The Guardian* newspaper (26 April 2008).

Beilock recruited a number of female university students to take a maths test. The women were divided into two groups. Before the test, the first group was told that the study was to understand why men, in general, do better than women at Maths. The aim of this question was to plant a seed of a stereotype in the mind of the participants. The second group was given no such information. When the results of the tests were analysed, they demonstrated that the group who were made aware of the stereotyping performed 10-15% worse than the other group.

When children have adopted a limiting belief based on negative feedback — perceived or actual — from parents or teachers, this will, in all probability, limit them. If the limiting belief is about intelligence or academic abilities, then performance in these areas will be impacted.

Unconscious bias

A negative view of a child could arise in many ways, one of which is unconscious bias. This refers to a bias that we are unaware of, and that happens outside our control. It happens automatically when our brain makes judgments and assessments of people and situations based on *our own* background, cultural environment, and personal experiences.

In the case of teachers, unconscious bias may manifest because of a child's colour or ethnicity. Likewise, parents may demonstrate unconscious bias when, for example, in a family of engineers, one child chooses to become an artist. In the eyes of the parents, although they love the child as much as their other children, the child may be considered in a more negative light.

Unfortunately, many cultures use vocation as a marker for intelligence. In such cultures, doctors, lawyers, engineers, and scientists are typically considered as highly intelligent and garner respect throughout the community. People in other vocations, however, may be viewed as being less intelligent.

A TEACHERS EXPECTATIONS INFLUENCES ACADEMIC PERFORMANCE

Numerous studies have proven that children perform better when their parents and teachers expect them to. Given these findings, parents need to be vigilant about the quality of teachers and the attitude that they have towards the children in their charge:

- If you have the option, choose a school in which teachers are known to believe in and have high aspirations for their students.

- Cultivate a relationship with your children in which they feel comfortable enough to openly discuss school matters with you.

- If there is any indication through discussion with your children, or from other parents, that a teacher has a negative view about your child, discuss the matter with the teacher.

- Draconian punishment, shaming, or talking down to a child, especially in front of their peers, should not be tolerated.

- At parent-teacher meetings, discuss the research that shows the importance of having a positive view of students.

8

The Importance of Mindset

"If parents want to give their children a gift, the best thing they can do is to teach their children to love challenges, be intrigued by mistakes, enjoy effort, and keep on learning. That way, their children don't have to be slaves of praise. They will have a lifelong way to build and repair their own confidence."

Carol Dweck, Professor of Psychology, Stanford University

The definition of mindset according to the Oxford English Dictionary is "The established set of attitudes held by someone". The foundation of all success — whatever the subject area — is mindset. Hard work, knowledge, effort, and persistence are important, but equally, if not more important, are the underlying beliefs and attitudes that form a person's mindset. This chapter talks about fixed mindsets and growth mindsets and why a growth mindset is what parents should be guiding their children towards.

Although children are not born with the belief that intelligence is fixed and invariable, in certain cultures, they eventually come to believe that it is.

In 1990 Stevenson and Lee discovered that whilst American mothers gave greater prominence to innate ability over effort, Chinese and Japanese mothers emphasised the importance of hard work over innate ability. The work of these researchers indicated that, in general, the Eastern Asian culture's recognition of the flexibility of intelligence and its emphasis on the role of **effort** promotes and embraces a lifelong **growth mindset**. On the other hand, the American culture, where the focus is on innate talent, gives rise to a **fixed mindset**.

In 2007, Kinlaw and Kurtz-Costes confirmed Stevenson and Lee's findings. Their data, published in *The Journal of General Psychology*, showed that in the USA, children are inclined to believe in the flexibility of intelligence until they are about half way through grade school. That is, they don't question whether intelligence can change over time. As they get older, however, their view changes and they start to see intelligence as fixed. They begin to believe that since their intelligence cannot change, their success or failure depends on circumstances outside their control, and, they end up with a **fixed mindset**.

The benefits of a growth mindset

Carol Dweck of Stanford University, through her twenty years of research, has demonstrated that what opens the doorways to success is a person's belief that they can become smarter and more talented. In her work, Dr Dweck demonstrated that people with a **fixed mindset** tend to shy away from challenges, give up easily, avoid hard work, respond badly to criticism, feel threatened by the success of others, and be more focused on proving intelligence.

In contrast to this, someone with a **growth mindset** enjoys challenges, accepts that hard work is required for success, overcomes hurdles, is inspired by the success of others, and does not strive to prove their intelligence.

As mentioned earlier, the way children are praised also affects their mindset. Research by Pomerantz and Kempner published in 2013 examined the effects on 120 children, comparing children who were praised for their intelligence rather than their effort. They found that when mothers praised a child for their intelligence, these children become more reluctant to tackle challenges due to fear of failure.

Even knowing about the growth mindset can produce results

Studies suggest that even becoming aware of the growth mindset can produce positive results. In a 2007 study by Blackwell et al, the researchers studied 7th graders and their achievement in Maths. Students were enrolled on one of two instructional programs. The first program taught children study skills — predominantly a **fixed mindset** approach. In the second program, children were given information about the brain as well as study tips. The second program encouraged children to see the brain as a muscle, a muscle that becomes stronger with use — a characteristic of a **growth mindset**.

The results showed that children enrolled in the second program (growth mindset) improved their maths grades whilst those that enrolled in the first program (fixed mindset) program did not.

Similar results are seen with college graduates. A study conducted by Niiya et al reported in *Psychological Science* (2004) selected two sets of college graduates with similar confidence in their academic abilities. The first group were primed with a theory that intelligence is fixed, whilst the second group were told that intelligence is variable. Compared to the second group, the first group experienced a higher level of negativity and lower self-esteem after suffering failure in an academic test.

Supporting students to adopt a growth mindset empowers children to accept more challenges, handle failure better, and learn from their mistakes.

Schroder et al published a paper in the journal *Biological Philosophy, (2014)* in which they demonstrated that simply reading a few short sentences about the differences between a growth mindset and a fixed mindset was enough to change the way students tackled a high-speed, attention-focused task. The students who were exposed to the "growth" mindset showed better focus and learned more from their mistakes when compared to students who read an endorsement of the fixed mindset.

Similarly, in a 2005 study by Thompson and Muskat, the researchers studied the puzzle solving abilities of students who initially had a fixed mindset. After they were informed about the growth mindset, their puzzle solving abilities improved.

A GROWTH MINDSET PRODUCES HIGH ACHIEVERS

A growth mindset promotes a focus on effort and produces high achievers. Achievers see that the key to getting ahead is not inherited talent or skill, but the result of hard work and effort. They believe that with effort and persistence, the intellect can be expanded and skills can be developed. This is the difference between the wildly successful and the merely mediocre.

- Tell children about the flexibility of the mind. Encourage them to view the brain as a muscle that gets stronger with more exercise.

- Teach them that the brain is a learning machine. Help them to understand that the brain learns by trying new things and by learning from mistakes. Encourage your children to view mistakes not as failures, but opportunities to learn – a part of the process towards success.

- The wrong kind of praise can backfire. Praising kids for being smart may encourage a fixed mindset. Praise children for the effort they put in, because this will promote a growth mindset.

9

Psychological Factors
that Influence IQ

*"It is not what you do for your children, but what you have taught them
to do for themselves, that will make them successful human beings."*

Ann Landers, American advice columnist

Self-confidence, self-esteem, self-worth, self-concept, and self-efficacy are all psychological terms that are sometimes confused as being the same. Although they are not the same, they are inter-related — albeit sometimes in complex ways. In this chapter, a few of these factors and their influence on intelligence will be examined, as well as motivation.

Self-esteem and self-worth

Both self-esteem and self-worth are measures of how much we value ourselves. Self-esteem comes from your feeling about yourself based on your actions and results compared to the world outside of you. Self-worth is deeper and comes from an inner knowing of your own intrinsic value. For the purposes of this book, and because many sources consider self-esteem and self-worth to be synonymous, we will consider them both as one and address them as "self-esteem".

Intuitively, one would expect a strong link between self-esteem and intelligence, however, the evidence is mixed. Some studies find a connection whilst others do not. Research that did uncover a connection includes the study by Simon and Simon. In 1975, Simon and Simon correlated self-esteem, intelligence, and academic achievement in a sample of 87 fifth graders and found a significant correlation between self-esteem and intelligence. Specifically, there was positive correlation between self-esteem and both verbal and nonverbal IQ, however, the association between verbal intelligence and self-esteem was stronger.

Other studies, however, found that self-esteem and intelligence were not related. For example, a 2015 study by Kaya and Oğurlu looked at the association between self-esteem, intelligence, and academic achievement. In a group of 127 middle school children, they found that there was no statistically significant relationship between self-esteem and intelligence.

In 1972, when Ronald Schnee studied 318 eighth grade and 478 fifth grade students, he found that IQ correlated significantly with all achievement subtests for the fifth graders, but not with self-esteem. Similarly, for eighth graders, IQ correlated with two of the maths subtests and self-esteem correlated with none. Math computation was the only factor related to self-esteem. In summary, Schnee found that bar this one exception, IQ and self-esteem are not related.

Although the evidence for a direct link between self-esteem and intelligence is mixed, err on the side of caution and help your child to develop high self-esteem

Self-confidence

Self-confidence is a person's belief in themselves and their abilities. According to behavioural geneticists Corina Greven and Robert Plomin, it is not just a state of mind but a genetic trait (this was explored in chapter 1).

Clinical psychologist Ann Reitan PsyD wrote a blog article in 2013 with the title *Child IQ – Why Confidence Matters*. In the article, she states that *"confidence and intellectual success reinforce each other. Any child who has confidence in his or her cognitive abilities will hypothetically score higher on IQ tests."* She goes on to say, *"Although many factors interact with genetic endowment to produce a child's intellectual capacity, the environmental component of intelligence is strong. In particular, confidence and cognitive association are hypothesized to be fundamental in formulating critical aspects of intelligence."*

In 2010, Sabina Kleitman from the University of Sydney published results of her research on self-confidence and its relationship to academic achievement in primary school children. She found a direct positive effect of self-confidence on achievement which holds true for both boys and girls of all ages. Kleitman's data clearly indicated that students who exhibit greater levels of self-confidence tend to perform better at school. Dhall and Thukral reported a similar positive relationship between self-confidence and intelligence in their sample of 1,000 students in Punjab, India.

In an article published in *Sex Roles* (2009), Steinmayr and Spinath investigated why boys have a stronger confidence in their intelligence than girls. In this paper, they *state "Following the logic of a self-fulfilling prophecy, thinking of oneself as inferior in ability might result in lower achievement when working on a test assessing that specific ability."* Chamorro-Premuzic et al (2010) verified this in their sample of 3,220 girls and 2,737 boys at ages 9 and 12. They found that self-perceived ability affects academic achievement. That is, the previous achievements of children affected their current self-perceived abilities in the form of a self-reinforcing, self-fulfilling prophecy.

> *Confidence or the lack of it can become a self-fulfilling prophecy. Confidence can lead to success, which leads to more confidence and greater success. It helps children to achieve greater academic success. Conversely, a lack of confidence can lead to failure, which further deflates confidence and can lead to further failure*

Self-concept and self-efficacy

Self-concept is how a person evaluates or perceives themselves, and self-efficacy is a person's perception and belief in their ability to complete tasks and reach goals. Self-efficacy is considered to be a subset of self-concept and most research is centred around self-concept.

In their 2016 paper, Svetlana D. Pyankovaa and Oksana V. Baskaevab state the widely-held view among psychologists that self-concept is the cornerstone of a child's development. Self-concept develops early and by the age of 4 or 5, a child can make self-evaluations. Many researchers have stated that academic self-perceptions play a key role in academic achievement because they enable students to develop their potential. The self-concept that students have of themselves influences learning and academic performance through, for example, processes such as increased effort and perseverance.

This connection between self-concept, learning and academic performance was explored by Hau and Kong in 1996. They studied the self-concept structure of 195 adolescent Chinese students' in many academic subjects and discovered a strong relationship between academic performance and self-concept.

Support for Hau and Kongs findings came from a paper in The American Journal of Nursing Science (2016). Hanan, Shabana, and Mona investigated the relationship between academic self-concept and students' performance among 182 school age children. Their findings indicated that there was a significant relationship between academic self-concept and students' performance. The researchers concluded that self-concept can impact intelligence, and the intelligence level, in its turn, can have an effect on self-concept.

How does motivation affect IQ?

Dr Angela Lee Duckworth of the University of Pennsylvania and her colleagues conducted a study that examined how much material incentives and motivation affected IQ scores. Their results were published in the *Proceedings of the National Academy of Sciences* (April 25, 2011, advance online edition).

They compared the IQ scores of test takers who had a material incentive with those who had no material incentive and discovered that motivation is a key component of performance in IQ tests. The results showed that everyone performs better with an incentive. Those who already had an above-average IQ to start with gained only 4 points when incentivised, whereas participants whose starting IQ was below average gained 16 points when incentivised.

Children may possess excellent cognitive ability, but lack the motivation to apply it. As a result, they will probably perform poorly on IQ tests and perhaps in their life as well. Boosting children's motivation will encourage them to put in the effort in to fulfil their potential.

A HIGH IQ IS BUILT ON PSYCHOLOGICAL WELL BEING

Confidence, self-esteem, self-worth, and self-concept are affected by relationships with caregivers that need to be strong, healthy, and positive. All other things being equal, a psychologically healthy child will be well positioned to succeed intellectually and in life.

Here are some ways to help your child increase their self-esteem and confidence:

- Encourage them to develop a sense of who they are.
- Praise them for their effort.
- Teach them to take pride in themselves and take good care of themselves.
- Guide them towards developing a healthy attitude to change.
- Give them the opportunity to make their own decisions.
- Encourage their aspirations — allow them to dream big dreams.
- Spend one-on-one time with them.
- Assign age-appropriate household chores.
- Don't do everything for them.
- Don't gush or offer insincere praise.
- Don't draw comparisons between them and their siblings or peers.
- Don't call them names or use sarcasm to make a point.
- Do improve your own self-confidence and self-esteem because you, as parents, are the ultimate role models for children.
- Motivate your children to fully exploit their talents and abilities. One of the best ways to do this is having a strong relationship with your child. Through that relationship, you can discover what motivates them.
- Appreciate them and accept them for who they are — complete with imperfections.

10

Encouraging Curiosity

"Curiosity is one of the permanent and certain characteristics of a vigorous intellect."

Samuel Johnson, lexicographer, poet, essayist and biographer

If you watch any baby or toddler, you will see their endless efforts to make sense of what they see and hear. They observe, imitate, poke, and prod to try to understand what things are and how they work. This is because we are all born curious. Unfortunately, the natural curiosity that we are born with is often cut short as we get older. In this chapter, we look at ways parents can ensure that this natural curiosity is not cut short but rather, nurtured to make it a lifelong habit.

In his 2014 Harvard Business Review article *"Curiosity Is as Important as Intelligence"*, Professor Tomas Chamorro-Premuzic, asserts that curiosity is one of the key psychological qualities that increase a person's ability to manage complexity. Curious people are more invested in developing their intellect and knowledge acquisition and their thinking style. Although Professor Chamorro-Premuzic makes a distinction between curiosity and intelligence, research has demonstrated that there is a correlation between curiosity and intelligence.

The *Journal of Personality and Social Psychology (2002)*, published a study in which investigators correctly predicted that later in life, more curious pre-schoolers would have higher IQs than less curious peers. Researchers evaluated the level of novelty-seeking behaviour in 1,795 children at age 3 and then, at age 11, they measured their cognitive ability. As forecasted, the highly curious 3 year olds scored 12 points higher in total IQ and had better academic achievement and reading ability at age 11 compared to the less curious 3 year olds. The work of Bornstein et al (2013) yielded similar results. They found that babies who explored more actively at 5 months achieved higher academic levels at age 14.

Other research supports the theory that exploration beginning in infancy contributes to long-term academic success. In fact, researchers Stumm et al published a paper in 2011 in which they propose that "intellectual curiosity is the third pillar of academic performance".

Curious children grow up to be smarter. Therefore, curiosity should be nurtured in children from a very early age. Studies on adults have shown that a high level of curiosity is connected to greater analytic ability, problem-solving skills, and overall intelligence.

As every parent knows, in recent times, schools have, become more test-driven, often at the expense of unstructured play. Susan Engel, author of *The Hungry Mind: The Origins of Curiosity in Childhood,* wrote in the *Harvard Education Review* (2011) that *"curiosity is both intrinsic to children's development and unfolds through social interactions. It should be cultivated in schools but is often almost completely absent from classrooms."*

Education Week, (2014) published an article by Erik Shonstrom in which he wrote that *"Students who do well in school are often curious or ambitious. I'd argue that the best learners — a term not necessarily synonymous with "best students" — have curiosity in abundance"*. He, like many other educators makes the point that the educational system is now so focused on testing and common curricula that there is very little room to nurture curiosity.

With the education system ever more focused on testing and rigid curricula, parents cannot rely on teachers to nurture curiosity. The onus is, therefore, on parents to cultivate their child's curiosity

CURIOSITY AND INTELLIGENCE GO HAND IN HAND

Curiosity is naturally present in children—it is a part of their makeup. As well as intelligence, curiosity correlates positively with health, social relationships, happiness, and meaning. Because it is such a desirable trait, parents and teachers should do everything within their power to allow curiosity to flourish. Here are some things you can do:

- Notice what captures your child's attention and imagination and encourage them to do more of the same. For example, if it's music, play it often, make and play instruments together, and dance together.

- Ask stimulating open-ended questions such as "What did you like about that book?" rather than "Did you like the book?"

- Create a safe yet interesting environment for your child to explore. Keep things fresh so they are constantly provided with new things to examine. When they come over to see what is happening or what you are doing, instead of marching them away, let them watch and observe from a safe vantage point.

- Allow them freedom and autonomy to explore their ideas and do what they want. One study showed how parents, by simply showing their children how to put together a model reduced the creative ways in which children could have accomplished this task. The moral is that it's better to let children figure things out by themselves.

❀ When a child is fascinated by something, quite often they will poke, prod, and pull apart that thing. Rather than stopping them or discouraging them, re-direct their attention to a similar alternative you have created for them. For example, if your toddler is persistently intrigued by your favourite plant and wants to pull off the leaves, rather than discouraging this, take them to a plant in area you have set up for them to explore.

❀ Children explore more when the adults they interact with model that type of behaviour. Be an adventurous family. Show your children that you enjoy being inquisitive. Show them that you don't know every answer, but you know how to find an answer when you don't know it.

11

Nurturing Creativity and Imagination

"Imagination is more important than knowledge. For knowledge is limited to all we now know and understand, while imagination embraces the entire world, and all there ever will be to know and understand."

Albert Einstein, physicist

Intelligence is classically defined as "the ability to acquire and utilise knowledge". Creativity, on the other hand is the ability to come up with new ideas through a process of mentally connecting existing concepts to arrive at new and novel solutions. Intelligence matters because it demonstrates the ability to gather knowledge and use it effectively. However, creativity goes beyond the frame of intelligence and has been called, by some, a higher order of intelligence.

Some studies of giftedness (an intellectual ability that is significantly higher than average) have shown that there is a clear relationship between high IQ and creativity. In 2005, Wai, Lubinksi, and Benbow published results showing that a high IQ is a predictor of creative achievement. But does this mean that activities which enhance a child's creativity will also increase IQ? It's a difficult question to answer quantitatively, but intuitively and subjectively, the answer is yes.

Wendy Masi PhD, dean of the Mailman Segal Institute of Childhood Studies at Nova Southeastern University in Fort Lauderdale and author of *Toddler Play*, says that "Nurturing creativity is one of the most important things you can do for your child". In fact, recent research indicates that a child's imagination quotient (described later in this chapter) may be a more important factor in predicting academic success than the more traditional measure of aptitude, the IQ score. "You want your child to be an original thinker, to understand that there isn't always one right answer to every situation," Dr Masi states.

Creativity, imagination, and intelligence go hand in hand. One of the greatest brains of the 20th century — Albert Einstein — was a keen proponent of using imagination. As well as the quote that opened this chapter, in a 1929 interview Einstein said, *"I am enough of the artist to draw freely upon my imagination. Imagination is more important than knowledge. Knowledge is limited. Imagination encircles the world"*. It is through imagination that creative ways of connecting existing concepts gives birth to innovation.

It is interesting to note that as well as being the creator of the Theory of Relativity, Albert Einstein played piano and violin. Thomas Edison played piano. Indeed, many scientists are creatives in their spare time. Einstein noted that "The greatest scientists are artists as well."

So, as schools place more emphasis on learning material and taking tests rather than creativity, there is concern from many quarters. Professor Rex Jung is concerned that opportunities for thoughts to flow freely and creatively are diminishing. Jung is a professor of neurosurgery at the University of New Mexico in Albuquerque, and together with others who study creativity, he asserts that creativity needs to be cultivated.

If you are interested in reading further into the relationship between creativity and intelligence, a good starting point is a 2015 paper published in the *Journal of Intelligence* by James Kaufman titled *Why Creativity Isn't in IQ Tests, Why it Matters, and Why it Won't Change Anytime Soon Probably*.

The Imagination Quotient (the other "IQ")

Given the important role that imagination played in the lives of people such as Einstein, it is somewhat of a surprise that it is not factored into the IQ test.

Dr Scott Barry Kaufman is a thought leader in the field of creativity and intelligence, and he is on a mission to correct this shortfall. During childhood, Dr Kaufman had a disorder that made it hard for him to process verbal information in real time. It took him longer to accomplish his tasks. This led him to be put into special education classes. In these classes, Kaufman was frustrated and felt unchallenged, but there wasn't much he could do. Fortunately, there was one teacher who sensed his frustration and decided to give him a test with no time limit. The results of the tests proved that Kaufman was capable of participating in normal classes and so he moved out of the special stream into the general stream. In his first semester in general classes, he went from a C-average to almost all As.

Later in life, he followed this success at school with a master's degree from Cambridge and a doctorate from Yale. He is now a Professor of Positive Psychology at the University of Pennsylvania and the Scientific Director of its Imagination Institute.

Kaufman believes that current IQ tests do a good job of evaluating general cognitive ability, but miss the many ways that ability interacts with engagement. *"In the school system, no one sees your inner stream of consciousness, your imagination. They only see how slow you are,"* he says. He is now working with other researchers to define and prepare tests to quantify an "imagination quotient". This imagination quotient will consider the many ways that imagination functions in people's work and maps what is going on in their brains.

CREATIVITY ENHANCES INTELLIGENCE

According to research, creativity, intelligence, and imagination are all related. However, quantifying the relationship is difficult. There are studies that have examined how high IQ inclines people towards creative endeavours, but there is little information about how creativity and imagination influence IQ.

Leading researchers emphasise the importance of taking steps to enhance the creativity and imagination of children. Some recommendations for parents and caregivers to enhance creativity and imagination are:

- ⚛ Give children permission to be different.
- ⚛ Let them disagree with you and express "divergent thought".

- ⚛ Encourage them to find more than one route to a solution.

- ⚛ Encourage play and process more than productivity.

- ⚛ Give young kids a diverse set of experiences to increase the chances of inspiration.

- ⚛ Limit TV and other screen time to make room for creative activities.

- ⚛ Encourage them to try, even though they may make mistakes. Failure is part of the process.

- ⚛ Provide the resources they need.

- ⚛ Celebrate innovation and creativity—display evidence of creative work around the house.

- ⚛ Avoid incentives where possible in creative endeavours. Unlike with tests, incentives can interfere with the creative process because the threat of missing the target makes it hard to innovate.

- ⚛ Allow children to master creative activities that they are instinctively motivated to do.

- ⚛ Let children be bored. Boredom challenges kids to engage with themselves and the world, to imagine, invent, and create. If they complain that they're bored, help them to come up with activities that would interest them. It's better they realise it's up to them to figure out how to make the best of their own time.

SECTION 3

NUTRITION, DIET, AND HEALTH

12

Junk Food and Anti-Nutrients

"Nourish the mind like you would the body. The mind cannot survive on junk food."

Jim Rohn, American entrepreneur and motivational speaker

As society is becoming more health conscious, more and more people are coming to understand that a diet predominantly made up of processed food — junk food — is bad for health. It can cause digestive problems, extreme fluctuations in blood sugar levels, diabetes, fatigue, weakness, depression, and many other problems. As well as these physical effects, science has shown that a junk food diet can have an impact on intelligence.

Fernando Gómez-Pinilla, a UCLA professor of neurosurgery and physiological science, has spent many years studying the effects of food, exercise, and sleep on the brain. His view on diet and the brain is that "food is like a pharmaceutical compound that affects the brain". Its influence is such that what your grandparents ate may have affected your parents and could now be influencing you and your abilities.

The link between diet, nutrition and IQ

Dr Lisa Smithers from the University of Adelaide led a study published in the *European Journal of Epidemiology* in 2012. The study showed that by the age of eight, children fed healthy diets had IQs up to 2 points higher than their counterparts who ate unhealthy food. Dr Smithers states, "While the differences in IQ are not huge, this study provides some of the strongest evidence to date that dietary patterns from six to 24 months have a small but significant effect on IQ."

In 2011, researchers from Bristol University wrote in the *Journal of Epidemiology and Community Health* that poor nutrition may affect brain development. Their study was based on the Avon Longitudinal Study of Parents and Children in which the eating habits of 3,966 children were recorded at the ages of 3, 4, 7, and 8½.

In the study, three types of diet were prominent: processed diets high in fat, sugar, and convenience foods; traditional diets of meat, potato, and vegetables; and health-conscious diets of salads, fruit, and fish.

The results showed that at the age of 3, a diet largely based on processed food was associated with a lower IQ at the age of 8½, irrespective of whether the diet improved after that age. In contrast, a healthy diet at age 3 was associated with a higher IQ at the age of 8 ½. The healthy diet, which is rich in fruits and vegetables, is nutritionally superior to a processed diet because of the abundance of important vitamins, minerals, plant chemicals, and fibre.

The work of Gale et al (2009) also confirmed the IQ advantages of a healthy diet. They conducted trials in developing countries to measure the effect of children's diet on their cognition and found that children whose diet in infancy was characterised by a high consumption of fruit, vegetables, and home-prepared foods had higher full-scale and verbal IQ and better memory performance aged 4.

> *If possible, freshly prepare food at home using as many vegetables as possible. Keep fruit readily available as a snack instead of sweets and crisps. If time or other constraints prevent you from cooking fresh food at home on most days of the week, you could cook a week's supply on one day and freeze it for use throughout the week. This is better than substituting home-prepared food with processed foods, which may be loaded with additives and preservatives.*

The effects of a poor diet

Sometimes, the effects of a poor diet can be noticed very quickly. A study published in 2015 in the journal *Nutrients* cites studies where it was found that *a single meal* with a high glycaemic load (a measure of the increase in blood glucose level after eating a meal) can impair memory performance in children and healthy young adults.

However, there is good news. Replacing a bad diet with a good diet can lead to better performance in a relatively short period of time as well. In 1986, Schoenthaler, Doraz, and Wakefield reported a 15.7% gain in academic performance for several hundred New York schools following the implementation of new diet policies that sharply lowered sugar, fat, and additive consumption.

Before the policy change, each child who ate the breakfast and lunch that the schools had always served scored relatively poorly on academic tests. After the policy change, once children started eating the new, nutritionally improved school breakfast and lunch, their academic scores improved. There was a clear link between the nutritional value of the food and academic scores. Furthermore, as more children ate the new healthy options, the overall achievement scores for the school improved.

School leaders take note: When you improve the nutritional quality of the meals served at your schools, any improvement in the academic scores of your students will reflect on the quality of your school.

Further proof that a poor diet affects learning comes from a study published in *Psychiatry Research* (Aug 2012). This study investigated the association between diet, attention-deficit disorder (ADD) and learning disabilities in school-aged children. Researchers discovered that when children with ADD and learning disabilities ate more nutrient-dense foods they paid more attention. Their learning and behaviour was better in school compared to children who ate more sweet, salty and fried foods.

When Dr Kate Northstone and Dr Pauline Emmett at The University of Bristol investigated the effects of overall diet on IQ at 8.5 years of age, they found that by the time they reached 8.5 years of age, 20% of the children who had the worst diet at the age of three had an IQ score 5 points lower, on average, than the group who ate the best diet. They scored quality of diet using a points system and in their paper, published in the *Journal of Epidemiology & Community Health*, (2011), they noted that every point increase in favour of a processed diet resulted in an IQ drop of 1.67 points. In contrast to this, a point increase towards a healthy diet resulted in an IQ gain of 1.2 points.

According to these researchers, brain growth occurs the fastest during the first three years of life, and therefore good nutrition during this period encourages optimal brain growth. The effect of a poor diet on brain development in these early years could persist forever, *even if the diet improves later.*

Although junk foods may contain many intelligence damaging ingredients, trans-fats are often one of the most vilified – for good reasons. First, they are a category of ingredient that is found in most processed foods, margarine, shortening, and fast foods – they are ubiquitous. Secondly, as researchers from the Oregon Health and Science University in Portland have demonstrated, trans-fats tend to take the place of healthy fats. This is a problem when it comes to the brain. The brain's normal signalling mechanism relies on healthy fats. When trans-fats steal the spots that are assigned to healthy fats the brain is compromised and performance is reduced.

Another consequence of poor diet is obesity. Obesity is a problem in many developed nations, and although some medical conditions can lead to obesity, it is usually caused by poor diet and lack of exercise. There is a negative association between intelligence and obesity, which has been well-established. A study published in *The Lancet* in 2014, states that amongst children and adolescents in developed countries, 23.8% of boys and 22.6% of girls were overweight or obese in 2013. Several past studies have correlated low IQ and obesity in children, however, it was only recently that the direction of causality was determined.

Satoshi Kanazawa's 2014 study demonstrated that low intelligence increases the chance of obesity. Does this imply that if parents work to increase their child's IQ they are also helping to reduce the likelihood of their child becoming obese? It could well be and certainly worthy of consideration.

Is ready-made baby food nutritionally adequate?

In the not-so-distant past, there was less reliance on processed food. Parents would prepare fresh food for their children and the food was nutritionally richer. Today, however, ready-made meals and processed baby foods are viewed by many overworked and overstressed parents as a quick and convenient way to feed their child. Although not all processed foods are harmful, many if not most of them, are high in sugar and artificial ingredients.

In 2013, Scientists from the Department of Human Nutrition at the University of Glasgow published a study in which they presented an analysis of all the baby foods produced by the main UK manufacturers. They found that many of these foods contained high levels of sugar. Also, because of these "fillers", babies would need to eat twice as much of this shop-bought food to get the equivalent amount of protein and energy as home-cooked meals. The researchers concluded that ready-made purees and spoon-able foods are generally much less nutrient-dense than homemade foods.

Other research has proven that some of the main brands are less nutritious than a cheeseburger (*The Guardian*, 2009). Such nutrient-deficient food is more harmful for babies than it is for adults because babies need nutrients more than they need calories. With processed food, there is a danger that babies will quickly fill up with empty calories, leaving them short of the nutrients that they need.

Researchers at the Greenwich University's School of Science examined the distribution of micro-nutrients in ready-made baby foods. They took eight different jars made by four major brands from the shelves of leading supermarkets and analysed them to determine the micro-nutrient content in each. The results, published in *Food Chemistry* (September 2011), revealed that the meals contained less than a fifth of the recommended daily intake of calcium, magnesium, zinc, iron, and other minerals.

Jars of food are convenient on the odd occasion especially when out and about, but the best option is for babies to eat food that is prepared at home. There are dozens of books packed with ideas for healthy, nutritious, and easy to prepare recipes for babies.

Foods to avoid

When thinking about foods to avoid, it's worth noting that some foods can attack IQ in more than one way. For example, sugar can have an immediate detrimental effect by interfering with blood sugar regulation and, in the longer term, it can lead to diabetes. Sugar can also lead to inflammation in the body. A team of Swedish scientists from the Karolinska Institute demonstrated that conditions such as inflammation are now being negatively associated with IQ.

In their 2010 paper published in *Brain, Behavior, and Immunity*, the Swedish researchers noted that *"Those with low-grade inflammation performed more poorly on standardised intelligence tests, even after excluding those with signs of current illness. Inflammation also predicted an increased risk of premature death."*

With this in mind, eliminating or limiting the consumption of the foods and ingredients listed below will, directly or indirectly, have a positive effect on IQ.

Refined carbohydrates: These are found in products made from processed white flour (white bread and pasta), cereals, crisps, and snacks. A diet high in refined carbs is likely to be low in selenium (a deficiency linked to irritability and depression), chromium (essential for blood-sugar control), zinc, iron, and B vitamins.

Professor Adrian Raine of the University of Southern California says that *"Poor nutrition characterised by zinc, iron, vitamin B, and protein deficiencies leads to low IQ, which leads to later antisocial behaviour. These are all nutrients linked to brain development."*

In Alexander Schauss's 1984 overview - *Nutrition and Behavior: Complex Interdisciplinary Research*, he presented a graph illustrating the degree to which carbohydrates affect IQ. The graph showed that when the carbohydrate content in a child's diet increased from 25% to 75%, their IQ dropped from nearly 110 points to just over 95 points.

In a 2013 article in *Psychology Today*, neurologist Dr David Perlmutter, described how consumption of carbohydrates elevates blood sugar in both the short and long term. To handle this additional blood sugar, the pancreas has to secrete more insulin. If the carbohydrate load persists, the eventual outcome will be insulin resistance. Insulin resistance may lead to dementia and type 2 diabetes. Type 2 diabetes is also associated with a doubling of the risk of developing Alzheimer's.

Citing from the from the *Journal of Alzheimer's Disease*, Dr Perlmutter states that people who favour carbohydrates in their diets increased their risk of developing dementia by 89% compared to those whose diets contained more fat than carbohydrates. Having the highest levels of fat consumption was found to be associated with a 44% *reduction* in the risk of developing dementia.

Carbohydrates are essential for good health however; refined carbohydrates are one of the worst foods for the brain and they should be avoided where possible.

Added sugars: Since the brain depends on glucose as its main source of energy, without enough glucose, brain performance will be affected. Therefore, there must be a source of glucose in our diet. This glucose can come from natural carbohydrates or natural sugars (such as the sugar in fruit) consumed as a part of a balanced diet. Added sugars, however, such as those added to sugary drinks, sweets, coated breakfast cereals, chocolate, and many other things not only impose an unnecessary burden on the body, but also have no nutritional value. As the body works hard to process the excess sugar, there can be a significant roller-coaster effect on alertness, concentration, and the ability to focus.

Dr Alex Richardson, a Senior Research Fellow at Oxford University, states *"If children slurp cans of sugary drinks on the way to school, it puts them on an artificial high in terms of brain function, but that stimulates the release of too much insulin which causes blood-sugar levels to plummet. In a short time, their brains are in a fog. They can't concentrate, they're irritable and find it hard to hold on to stable emotional reactions."*

Fried foods: Fried or processed foods contain trans-fats, additives, preservatives, and many other chemicals. Our brains rely on natural fats to create and maintain cell membranes and carry fat-soluble vitamins. Trans-fats, on the other hand, are chemically-altered fats that can cause cellular destruction, upset hormone production, increase inflammation in the brain, and have a detrimental effect on memory.

Artificial sweeteners: Artificial sweeteners are found in diet sodas and processed foods labelled "sugar-free". They are marketed as a means to get the sweetness of sugar without the calories. However, they are not the panacea they are often made out to be.

A 2013 post in *Psychology Today* titled *Just Say "no" to Artificial*

Sweeteners states that *"People who consume 'light' drinks and foods usually do so for weight loss, or to prevent weight gain. Several epidemiological studies, however, have shown that the opposite is true: not only do they not aid in weight-loss, they actually stimulate appetite and promote weight gain!"*

In addition, a 2009 study by Nettleton et al published in *Diabetes Care* concluded that artificial sweeteners increase the risk of insulin resistance. People who drink a diet soda daily have a 36% greater chance of developing the metabolic syndrome (insulin resistance syndrome) and a 67% increased risk of type 2 diabetes.

The European Journal of Clinical Nutrition (August 2007) published a study in which researchers examined the effects of the artificial sweetener aspartame on the brain. They reported that prenatal consumption of aspartame might result in mental retardation. Additionally, this sweetener is implicated in disrupting learning and emotional functioning due to its involvement in altering certain neurotransmitters and might affect early brain development.

Dr Russell Blaylock, in his 1998 book *Excitotoxins: The Taste that Kills,* states that *"Nutrasweet (Aspartame) has been scientifically linked to brain tumours, brain cell damage and neurological conditions such as Alzheimer's and Parkinson's disease."*

Beyond this, artificial sweeteners have been implicated as contributors to: brain fog, migraines, dizziness, anxiety, depression, impaired vision, and increasing symptoms of ADHD.

Saturated fats: Saturated fats have long been vilified by the medical community and the media. This was primarily because early in the 20th century, researchers found that eating saturated fats raised cholesterol and they linked the increase in cholesterol to heart disease. However, new research has identified that it is carbohydrates, certain fats, and inflammation which are the main contributors to heart disease.

In fact, Dr David Perlmutter states that *"saturated fat is a fundamental building block for brain cells. It's certainly interesting to consider that one of the richest sources of saturated fat in nature is human breast milk."*

The importance of cholesterol to the correct functioning of the brain is such that 25% of the body's cholesterol is found in the brain. Cholesterol protects the brain through its antioxidant properties, provides the raw material that our bodies use to make vitamin D, and it is the forerunner to three hormones that contribute to brain health - oestrogen, progesterone, and testosterone.

Since the brain is mainly made of fat and cholesterol, saturated fats are good for the brain. But what if there is too much saturated fat in our diet? A study published in 2016 by Dr Kevin Woollard and colleagues at Imperial College London concluded that a diet containing high levels of saturated fat promotes inflammation and tissue damage. Too much fat, like too much of anything, is not healthy. However, as long as your diet is balanced, saturated fats are not considered to be as bad as they were previously thought to be.

Trans-fats: There are, broadly speaking, two types of trans fats found in foods. One type is naturally occurring and the other type is artificial. The natural variety is created in the stomach of some animals and foods derived from these animals. Products such as milk and meat products may contain small amounts of these fats.

The artificial variety (also known as trans fatty acids) are manufactured by combining hydrogen with liquid vegetable oils. Trans-fats in processed food are usually labelled as "partially hydrogenated oils". This type of trans fat should be avoided as it's known to trigger systemic inflammation, raise bad (LDL) cholesterol levels, and lower good (HDL) cholesterol levels.

Trans-fats deprive the brain of oxygen by clogging veins and arteries. Furthermore, they rob the brain of the essential chemical apolipoprotein E, which hinders the regulation of amyloids which leads to abnormal neuron function.

Omega-6 fatty acids: The body needs a balance of omega-6 and omega-3 fatty acids. However, too much omega-6 can trigger the body to produce pro-inflammatory chemicals as described in the paper *Health Implications of High Dietary Omega-6 Polyunsaturated Fatty Acids published in the Journal of Nutrition and Metabolism (2012).* The main offenders, as far as omega-6 fatty acids are concerned, are: corn oil, safflower oil, sunflower oil, grapeseed oil, soy oil, peanut oil, vegetable oil, mayonnaise, and many salad dressings.

Gluten and casein: Some people are intolerant to gluten and casein (proteins found in dairy and wheat). The intolerance affects the lining of the small intestine and can have a drastic effect on academic performance.

In 2010, Dr David Perlmutter wrote an article in *the Huffington Post* in which he discussed the case of a nine-year-old girl who had significant issues with her academic performance. At times, she was fine, but at other times she had difficulty thinking and focusing and was falling behind with her school work. When tested for food sensitivities, she was discovered to be profoundly sensitive to gluten. Her parents immediately eliminated all wheat, barley, and rye from her diet and within two weeks, there was a marked improvement in her cognitive function

Diacetyl: Most of the diacetyl that is consumed is in processed foods, where it is added to provide a rich, buttery flavour. The American Chemical Society published the results of a study in August 2012 stating that diacetyl intensifies the damaging effects of an abnormal brain protein linked to Alzheimer's disease. It is the main flavouring agent used in margarine, shortening, oil sprays, and many butter substitutes. Diacetyl is also present in microwave popcorn, potato chips, corn chips, crackers, biscuits, and desserts. The label may not have the word diacetyl on the label, but look out for "artificial butter flavour" or "natural flavours".

Monosodium glutamate (MSG): MSG is an excitotoxin — a substance that overexcites cells to the point of damage. Many high-fat carbohydrate and high sugar foods contain MSG, which makes them taste better. However, the price of this better taste can be expensive, since early exposure to MSG damages brain cells in the hypothalamus, which regulates the hormones for growth, reproduction, and sleep.

In 1968, Dr Olney from the Department of Psychiatry at Washington University in St. Louis studied the effects of MSG. He found that it leads to retinal destruction and widespread destruction of the neurons to the hypothalamus and other adjacent areas of the brain.

Neuroscientist and author Dr Russell Blaylock has written extensively about the dangers of MSG and its potential to damage the brain. He states that children are four times more sensitive to excitotoxins than adults. The effects of excitotoxin damage during the formative years from 1 week after conception to the age of six or seven can have profound health implications. With regard to intelligence, hyperactivity, lack of focus, and lowered intelligence have all been observed in animal studies.

If you want more information about the damaging effects of MSG and Aspartame, Dr Blaylock's 1998 book *Excitotoxins: The Taste that Kills* is recommended reading. Alternatively, a short Kindle book *The Truth About Aspartame, MSG and Excitotoxins – an interview with Dr Russell Blaylock by Mike Adams* provides a very concise but useful summary.

Synthetic food colours: In 2007, *The Lancet* published the results of a study by the University of Southampton where it was concluded that some colouring additives lowered children's IQ by up to 5 points. As a result of these findings, the UK's Food Advisory Service imposed a voluntary ban on the use of these colourings by the UK food industry. Many food manufacturers complied but some have yet to comply. The colourings in question are: quinoline yellow (E104), sunset yellow (E110), carmoisine (E122), allura red (E129), tartrazine (E102), and ponceau 4R (E124).

KEEP CHILDREN AWAY JUNK FOOD

Junk food and the many ingredients that are used to impart flavour and body to junk food are directly or indirectly detrimental to IQ. However, some of the ingredients in junk food are required by the body – in measured doses, for example, sugar and carbohydrates. The body *does* need sugar and it *does* need carbohydrates and many of the other compounds discussed in this chapter, however, they are only useful in the appropriate quantities.

Your aim should be to fulfil your child's dietary requirements with *appropriate amounts* of natural foods, rather than processed and chemically altered foods. Over time, replace as many processed foods with an *appropriate amount* of fresh, natural food as possible. However, be careful not to jump to the other extreme. For example, eliminating processed sugar is a good strategy, but doubling the overall sugar intake through eating more sugar-rich fruits will still flood the body with more sugar than it needs. Strive for balance.

The body has a remarkable ability to adapt to, and cope with, many stressors. Occasional and limited indulgence in junk food will most likely have little impact on IQ or health, but junk food can become addictive. Habitually eating "bad" food can lead to irreversible changes in mind and body performance. So, as far as possible, eliminate or strictly limit the following:

- Processed foods
- Refined carbohydrates
- Foods with added sugars
- Artificial sweeteners
- Additives and synthetic food colours

13

Foods, Vitamins, and Minerals That Boost Brainpower

"We do children an enormous disservice when we assume that they cannot appreciate anything beyond drive through fare and nutritionally marginal, kid-targeted convenience foods. Our children are capable of consuming something that grew in a garden or on a tree and never saw a deep fryer. They are capable of making it through dinner at a sit-down restaurant with tablecloths and no climbing equipment. Children deserve quality nourishment."

Victoria Moran, author and inspirational speaker

To function effectively, the brain needs an adequate supply of vitamins and minerals. When there is a nutritional deficiency, neuron signals may slow down and the membranes that protect brain cells from damage can deteriorate. This affects children's' health, behaviour, and ability to think. Ideally, all the nutrients that the brain needs should come from a balanced diet. A balanced, nutritionally-rich diet leads to better exam performance, higher scores in Maths, increased attendance, and better overall academic performance. In the first part of this chapter, some of the foods that are associated with good brain function will be summarised. The second part discusses vitamins and minerals. Implementing the suggestions in this chapter can help improve your child's IQ.

What are antioxidants and why are they important?

Before we discuss foods, vitamins, and minerals, it is useful to say a few words about free radicals and antioxidants.

The cells in your body are constantly under attack, and one of the ways they are attacked is through free-radical damage. Free-radicals are unattached oxygen molecules that attack cells in the way that oxygen causes metal to rust. You can see this effect when you cut an apple or peel a banana. After a short while, you will see the fruit turn brown – this is damage caused by oxygen. Antioxidants attach to free radicals, rendering them harmless.

So how does this affect IQ? In the body, free radicals attack cells, and this causes cells to lose their ability to function properly, and eventually they die. The brain uses a lot of oxygen — about 20% of all the oxygen that you breathe. This means that brain cells are particularly vulnerable to free-radical damage because of the amount of oxygen the brain uses.

Children who eat a nutrient-dense diet are providing their brains with supplementary antioxidant support, which helps to protect against free-radical attacks.

Foods that are associated with better brain function

In the following paragraphs, you'll find a list of many foods containing nutrients that benefit the brain.

Fruit: Fruit not only tastes great, but together with vegetables, it provides many of the nutrients that the brain needs to develop and function effectively. Nutritionists recommend eating at least 5-7 portions of a variety of vegetables and/or fruit every day.

Vitamin C is one nutrient that is abundant in fruit. As well as being an antioxidant, vitamin C is also good for IQ, as the following study demonstrates.

Jean Carper, the author of *Your Miracle Brain,* referred to a 1960 study undertaken by researchers at Texas Woman's University who tested the IQ and vitamin C levels of 236 school children and 115 university students. They found that students with the highest vitamin C levels had IQ scores that were 5-10 points higher than students with the lowest levels of vitamin C.

When the students were given orange juice at school for six months, the IQ of the students with low vitamin C levels increased by around four points. The students with originally high vitamin C levels improved very little in their IQ scores. Carper wrote that *"IQ scores generally rose along with blood vitamin C concentrations."*

However, vitamin C is water-soluble and because of this, the body doesn't store it well. As a result, foods rich in vitamin C need to be consumed every day.

Berries are also ideal fruits as they contain all of the IQ-enhancing benefits of vitamin C, plus they are packed with antioxidants. Seeds from berries also contain omega-3 fats that help with brain function. The more intense the colour of the berry, the more nutritional power it has. Encourage your children to eat strawberries, cherries, blueberries, and blackberries.

There is one caveat with fruit: because they are rich in sugar, you should take care to balance fruit intake with vegetables. Be careful not to overdo fruit consumption.

Vegetables: Feed your children a variety of vegetables that are diverse in flavours and colours. This helps to provide a broad a range of nutrients and vitamins. All leafy vegetables are rich in vitamin B9 (folates). Many vegetables such as tomato, eggplant, pumpkin, sweet chili, and corn also contain antioxidants that help restore damaged cells.

Protein-rich foods: Protein increases the concentration of dopamine, which is a brain chemical associated with mental alertness. Dr Judith Wurtman of the Massachusetts Institute of Technology in America recommends the best foods to eat just before an event that requires maximum concentration are fish, shellfish, skinless chicken, and egg white, which are high in protein and low in fat. Parents should keep this is mind when their children are preparing for major events at school that require focus and concentration.

A few protein sources for vegetarians and vegans include green peas, tofu, nuts, chickpeas, edamame, beans, broccoli, chia seeds, and Quorn.

Oily fish: Over 65% of the fatty acids that belong to the omega family make up more than half of our brain mass. Omega-3 and omega-6 fats are vital to the production and development of brain cells. They also play a huge role in neuron activity.

Scientists from the United States National Institutes of Health studied data from a long-term research project in Avon, UK. They found that in a group of 9,000 mothers and their children, the children of mothers with the smallest intake of Omega-3 had a verbal IQ that was 6 points lower than the average.

Both omega-3 and omega-6 fats are essential, but omega-6 causes inflammation. Also, since both fats compete with each other, how can we ensure that the right balance is achieved?

The typical modern western diets have omega-6 to omega-3 ratios between 15:1 to 17:1. Experts say that we should default to the diet our ancestors ate, where the ratio of omega-6 to omega-3 was 1:1.

Vegetarians and vegans can increase their Omega-3 intake through many supplements currently available online or in health food shops. The Vegetarian Society factsheet on omegas lists green leafy vegetables such as lettuce, broccoli, kale, purslane, and spinach as sources of omega-3. Nuts and legumes such as mungo, kidney, navy, pinto, or lima beans, peas, or split peas are also good sources.

Eggs: Eggs are rich in protein, vitamins, and minerals, all of which play a very important part in a child's development. Additionally, eggs also contain DHA (docosahexaenoic acid — an omega-3 fatty acid) and lecithin, both of which stimulate the development of the nervous system and the body, and positively affect the development of the brain. Eggs are also rich in choline, which is beneficial for memory.

Although choline is good for memory, too much is known to become carcinogenic. For this reason, it is recommended that adults have no more than two eggs per day. To determine the healthy maximum for your children, it would be wise to consult a nutritionist.

Oysters: Oysters are a good source of the mineral zinc, which can help with learning and memory. Zinc also helps detoxify heavy metals including lead, which is one of the biggest environmental threats to IQ.

Milk and yoghurt: Dairy products are a good source of B vitamins, which are essential for the growth of brain cells, neurotransmitters, and enzymes. Low-fat milk and yoghurt are also great sources of vitamin D, protein, and carbohydrates, all of which the brain needs to function optimally.

For vegans or those who are dairy-intolerant, there are numerous plant-based sources of B vitamins. Vitamin D is also produced by the body from sunlight. In addition, D and B vitamins are available as supplements.

Pulses, lentils, peas, and beans: Pulses are a cheap, low glycaemic index, low-fat source of protein, fibre, vitamins, and complex sugars. The brain is dependent on glucose — it consumes more than 5 grams per hour. Because it cannot store glucose, it needs a constant supply. Pulses help to keep blood sugar levels stable, which keeps the brain supplied with this vital fuel. Much of intellectual performance depends on the blood level of glucose.

Nuts and seeds: Nuts are a great snack. They are a good source of protein, vitamin E (which protects brain cell membranes from free radical damage), and omega-3 and omega-6 fats, both of which are crucial to brain and eye development.

Water/hydration: Up to 60% of the human adult body is water. According to H.H. Mitchell in the *Journal of Biological Chemistry*, the brain and heart are composed of 73% water, so it's understandable why not drinking enough water has a detrimental effect on our brains. When your body lacks water, brain cells and other neurons shrink, and biochemical processes involved in cellular communication can slow down.

Water is great for memory sharpness and helps to keep your mood stable. Dehydration makes children listless, lethargic, and irritable. Ensure that your children drink plenty of water and snack on high water-content foods such as cucumber, watermelon, carrots, celery, and tomatoes.

Anti-inflammatory foods: In a study conducted by a team of Swedish scientists from the Karolinska Institute in Stockholm, researchers noted that participants in the study who had low-grade inflammation performed more poorly on standardised intelligence tests.

There is a lot of information on anti-inflammatory foods and ingredients online, but here's a short list:

- **Vegetables**: Green leafy vegetables, celery, beets, broccoli, blueberries.
- **Fruits**: Pineapple, tomatoes, blueberries, strawberries, raspberries.
- **Spices**: Turmeric, ginger.
- **Seeds and nuts**: Chia seed, flaxseeds, walnuts, almonds.
- **Oils**: Coconut oil, olive oil.

You will notice that this list of foods contains many of the "brain food" ingredients listed earlier.

Foods that have been known to cause inflammation should be taken in moderation include: dairy products, sugar, refined carbohydrates, meat, and artificial trans fats.

Should you supplement your child's diet with minerals and vitamins?

The *Journal of the American College of Nutrition, December 2004* reported that between 1950 and 1999, the nutritional value of our fruits and vegetables had significantly declined. Lead author Dr Donald Davis said that 6 out of 13 nutrients showed declines ranging from 6% to 38%.

Given these findings and the modern western diet, which is often nutritionally unbalanced, it may be useful to add vitamin and mineral supplements to your child's daily regimen. This is especially true if your child is on a restricted diet, such as vegan, or if there are health issues that affect their absorption of nutrients. Before you supplement your child's diet, however, it is worth getting advice from a certified nutritionist or medical practitioner.

The following studies indicate the degree to which supplementing a child's food intake with vitamins and minerals can affect IQ.

Stephen Schoenthaler, a professor at California State University at Stanislaus, and his colleagues tested the IQs of 245 schoolchildren between the ages of 6 and 12 in Phoenix, Arizona. After testing, they enlisted teachers to distribute either a vitamin and mineral supplement or a placebo to the children on a daily basis. The results, published in 2000, demonstrated that students who were given the supplements during the course of the study had an average *2.5-point gain in IQ*. Those children who were poorly nourished at the start of the study *gained 15 or more IQ points* by the end of the study.

The researchers also noted that test scores were closely linked with school performance, and they suggested that parents *"of schoolchildren whose academic performance is substandard would be well advised to seek a nutritionally oriented physician for assessment of their children's nutritional status"*.

In an earlier study (1988), Dr David Benton and Gwilym Roberts supplemented the diet of 60 school children with a combination of multi-vitamins and minerals designed to provide the ideal level of essential nutrients. Benton and Roberts found that after eight months of supplementation, the non-verbal IQs of the children increased by 9 points.

Poor nutrition — especially in early life — can have an impact much later in life, as indicated by a study published in the *British Medical Journal* (November 1998). In the study, 424 premature babies were split into two groups. For one month after birth, one group was fed a "nutrition-enriched" pre-term formula milk whilst the second group were fed a standard formula. At age 8, boys on the pre-term formula had a 12.2 point advantage in verbal IQ and a 6.3 point advantage in overall IQ over those fed the standard formula. The researchers stated that IQ at this age is highly predictive of IQ in adults, suggesting that bad nutrition in the early years can have a permanent effect on ability.

Which vitamins and minerals supplements help to boost IQ?

There are specific vitamins and minerals supplements that are conducive to better brain functioning. They fulfil a variety of roles, for instance, some help to ensure the health of neurons (nerve cells). Others are needed to manufacture neurotransmitters (brain chemicals that transmit information through the brain).

B vitamins, in particular, play important roles in children's brain development. Deficiencies in B vitamins can cause problems with learning, focusing, and memory.

In 2008, *Nature Reviews: Neuroscience* listed the following possible brain-related outcomes of deficiencies in certain B vitamins:

- A folate deficiency during childhood affects brain function even into adulthood.

- A thiamine deficiency can cause a numbing effect on brain nerves.

- A riboflavin deficiency may lead to brain dysfunction.

- A niacin deficiency may cause memory loss.

- A vitamin B-12 deficiency can lead to brain deterioration and delayed development.

The following table lists the vitamins that are associated with brain health and the foods that supply them. You can supply the various nutrients to your children through individual supplements or through the many food sources listed:

Vitamin	Role in Brain Health	Food Source
Vitamin A	Increases the brain's ability to form new neurons and is critical to memory and wakefulness.	Sweet potatoes, carrots, dark leafy greens, winter squashes, lettuce, dried apricots, cantaloupe, bell peppers, fish, liver, and tropical fruits.
Vitamin B1 (thiamine)	Required for the manufacture of some neurotransmitters and normal nerve function.	Pork, ham, dark green leafy vegetables, fortified whole-grain cereals and baked goods, wheat germ, enriched rice, green pea, lentils, and nuts such as almonds and pecans.

Vitamin	Role in Brain Health	Food Source
Vitamin B2 (riboflavin)	Maintains healthy blood cells and helps to boost energy levels.	Milk and milk products such as yoghurt and cheese; asparagus, spinach, and other dark green leafy vegetables; chicken, fish, eggs, and fortified cereals.
Vitamin B3 (niacin)	Is particularly useful for enhancing memory.	Chicken, turkey, salmon, and other fish including canned tuna packed in water. Fortified cereals, legumes, peanuts, pasta, and whole wheat also supply varying amounts.
Vitamin B4 (choline)	Stimulates production of acetylcholine, which is responsible for memory, mental clarity, and the connections between neurons.	Eggs, liver, peanuts, meat, poultry, fish, dairy foods, pasta, rice, spinach, beets, wheat, and shellfish.
Vitamin B5 (pantothenic acid)	Helps to improve memory and mental alertness.	Yoghurt, sweet potatoes, legumes including lentils and split peas, avocado, mushrooms, and broccoli.
Vitamin B6 (pyridoxine)	Required for neurotransmitter manufacture and converting amino acids into the important neurotransmitter serotonin.	Poultry, seafood, bananas, potatoes, fortified cereals, and leafy green vegetables such as spinach.
Vitamin B9 (folic acid)	Essential for oxygen delivery to the brain.	Dark green vegetables such as broccoli, spinach, collard or turnip greens, okra, Brussels sprouts, and asparagus. Avocado, lentils, dried beans, peas, nuts, citrus fruit, and juice.

Vitamin	Role in Brain Health	Food Source
Biotin	Required to produce myelin, which is an important part of the nervous system and vital for cognitive function	Egg yolks, liver, salmon, avocado, pork. Most fruits, vegetables, cheeses, and grains contain a little biotin.
Vitamin B12	Particularly important for infants. A deficiency may slow down a baby's physical and mental development and cause nerve damage.	The only natural source is animal foods — shellfish, such as clams, mussels and crab, fin fish, and beef. Vegetarians and vegans can find this in in soy products and cereals, which are fortified with B12.
Vitamin C	Regulates neurotransmitter systems of the brain and aids the general development and health of neurons.	Peppers, guavas, mangos, citrus fruits, berries, broccoli, kiwi fruit, peas, papaya, pineapple, and watermelon.
Vitamin D	Aids the development of the brain and nervous system.	Sunshine. Fish oils, fatty fish, mushrooms, beef liver, cheese, and egg yolks.
Vitamin E	Has antioxidant effects and promotes concentration, precision, and clarity.	Almonds, raw seeds, swiss chard, mustard greens, spinach, turnip greens, kale, plant oils, hazelnuts, broccoli, parsley, papaya, and olives.

Vitamin	Role in Brain Health	Food Source
Vitamin K	Research on this is in the early stages, but it has been observed to sharpen memory in older adults. Its role in cognition is still being investigated.	Collards, green leaf lettuce, kale, mustard greens, parsley, romaine lettuce, spinach, Swiss chard, turnip greens, broccoli, Brussels sprouts, cauliflower, and cabbage. To a lesser degree, meats, fish, liver, eggs, and cereals.

Mineral	Role in Brain Health	Food Sources
Chromium	Enhances cognition.	Whole grains, bread, brown rice, broccoli, mushrooms, green beans, brewer's yeast, beef, beer, chicken, cheese, eggs, fish, sea food, corn, potatoes, dairy products, and fresh vegetables.
Magnesium	Improves learning and memory functions.	Raw spinach, mackerel, nuts and seeds, beans and lentils, whole grains, and avocado.
Zinc	Low zinc levels have been associated with reduced learning ability, apathy, lethargy, and mental retardation.	Toasted wheat germ, spinach, pumpkin seeds, squash seeds, nuts, dark chocolate, pork, chicken, beans, mushrooms, oysters, beef, and lamb.
Iron	Important for cognitive function and development. Iron deficiency has been found to lead to lower IQ, and poor thinking and problem-solving abilities in children.	Meat and seafood, leafy greens, nuts, and beans, as well as foods fortified with iron such as cereal, bread, and pasta.

Mineral	Role in Brain Health	Food Sources
Iodine	Deficiency leads to mental retardation.	Sea vegetables, cranberries, yoghurt, strawberries, cheese, potatoes.
Bioflavonoids	Antioxidants that prevent cell damage.	Red bell peppers, strawberries, citrus fruits, broccoli, brussels sprouts, tropical fruits, garlic, spinach, green tea.
Omega-3	Can promote brain health by facilitating enhanced communication between brain cells.	Flaxseed oil, fish oil, chia seeds, walnuts, oysters, soy beans, spinach.

Does organic food help to increase IQ?

Before the advent of mass farming, food was grown without the use of chemical fertilizers and pesticides. Today, many pesticides such as fungicides, herbicides, and insecticides are widely used in conventional agriculture. As discussed in the chapter "Toxins", research clearly shows that many chemicals are neurotoxic and have a detrimental effect on the IQ of children.

According to the American Academy of Pediatrics (AAP), children are most commonly exposed to toxins through pesticide residues on food. In October 2012, in a report published in *Pediatrics*, the AAP stated that an organic diet undoubtedly reduces exposure to pesticides and that it may also decrease the incidence of diseases associated with a resistance to antibiotics.

School-age children have lower IQs when their mothers are exposed to pesticides during pregnancy. One study titled *Prenatal Exposure to Organophosphate Pesticides and IQ in 7-Year-Old Children* found that children whose mothers-to-be had the highest concentrations of the pesticide dialkyl phosphate in their body during pregnancy had an average deficit of 7.0 IQ points at age 7.

Because organic food is exposed to fewer toxic pesticides, it can help to minimise IQ loss attributable to toxins.

NOURISH THE MIND TO INCREASE IQ

A good diet during childhood not only provides nutritional support for the brain, but it may establish lifelong dietary habits that will have a positive effect on a child's intelligence and overall health throughout life.

Here are some guidelines to follow:

- If you feel unsure about the level of nutrition that your child needs, consult a nutritionist.

- You child should eat a good mix of fruit and vegetables every day — 5 to 7 portions in total.

- Set an example by eating healthy yourself — be a role model for your kids.

- Make a variety of healthy foods and snacks available at home. When the inevitable desire for a snack arises, your children have the choice to opt for healthy snacks rather than junk food.

- Make sure that your children are hydrated throughout the day.

- At mealtimes, serve water instead of soft drinks.

- Involve your children in food shopping and preparing meals. This is a great opportunity to teach your children about nutrition, provide them with a feeling of accomplishment, and may even make them more willing to eat or try foods that they help prepare.

- Choose organic foods where possible. If you have the opportunity, grow your own food.

14

The Breakfast Advantage

"One should not attend even the end of the world without a good breakfast."

Robert A. Heinlein, American science-fiction writer

The adage that breakfast is the most important meal of the day is now supported by Science. Evidence shows that there are many health benefits associated with breakfast. Breakfast is particularly important for children because it has been proven to lead to improved concentration, attention span, memory, and a higher IQ.

An article published by the United Nations University (January 2013) presented research that measured IQ and its relationship with the nutritional status and breakfast intake habits of 529 primary school children in Baghdad, Iraq. The results of the study revealed a clear relationship between IQ and consumption of breakfast. Compared with a control group, the risk of having low intelligence was shown to be 11.6 times greater for malnourished children and 7.4 times greater for children who skip breakfast. In terms of IQ, there was a 4.69-point decrease in children who skip breakfast and 7.3-point decrease in malnourished children. Also noted was a 3.2 point drop in IQ when children's nutritional habits were poor.

Dr Jianghong Liu and fellow researchers also found that poor breakfast habits impacted children's IQs. The children in their cohort were 1,269 six-year-olds in China. Their paper, published in 2013, reported that children who did not have breakfast regularly had verbal IQ and total IQ scores that were 5.58 points and 4.6 points lower, respectively, than children who regularly ate breakfast.

Other researchers have suggested that the sort of breakfast that children eat and how regularly they have breakfast both have an impact on IQ. For example, low glycaemic index foods such as oats are associated with better learning because they do not cause an initial spike in blood glucose after they are consumed.

In 2005, Mahoney and colleagues published the results of a study examining the effects of three types of breakfast on elementary children's scores in cognitive tests. The different breakfast options were: ready-to-eat cereal, instant oatmeal, or no breakfast.

Their results showed that among children aged 9 to 11, eating either cereal or oatmeal improved cognitive performance relative to no breakfast. However, oatmeal was more beneficial than ready-to-eat cereal because oatmeal improved spatial memory in both boys and girls. For girls, it also enhanced short-term memory. Both spatial ability and memory are attributes that are measured in IQ tests. When younger children aged 6 to 8 were studied, the same results were noted. The younger children also demonstrated improved auditory attention.

A study by Herrero et al published in *Nutricion Hospitalari* (May 2006) showed that an increase in the quality of breakfast (e.g. breakfast containing ingredients from each of the main food groups) led to a significant increase in students' average grades at the end of the year.

REGULAR BREAKFAST BOOSTS IQ

Breakfast has a big impact on a child's IQ and academic performance. Parents and schools should encourage children to eat breakfast regardless of the food choice, since any breakfast is better than no breakfast.

- If there is a choice, then lower glycaemic index breakfast foods (such as oatmeal) and a complete breakfast that includes a few different food groups are better.

- Regular high-quality breakfasts will help a child to achieve better grades at school.

- There are many excellent breakfast recipes online that are quick and easy to prepare. Some examples include:

  - Low-fat bio-yoghurt topped with whole grain cereal and fruit.
  - Vegetable omelette and milk.
  - Tomato, avocado, and cheese on whole wheat toast.
  - Whole grain, low-sugar cereal with milk and a piece of fruit.
  - Steel-cut oatmeal with sliced apples, cinnamon, and nuts.
  - A piece of string cheese, a piece of fruit, and a handful of pumpkin seeds.

15

Toxins

"Cells depend on chemical signals to tell them where to go, how to connect, and which genes to turn on or off. Any foreign substance that interferes with the clear transmission of these chemical messages can impact negatively on development."

Thomas J Darvill, PhD, Chairman of Psychology,
Oswego State University, New York.

Multiple studies illustrate that lower IQs directly correlate to early chemical exposure in children. The evidence is strong that even extremely low levels of exposure to toxic metals, such as lead and mercury, and persistent toxins, such as polychlorinated biphenyl (PCBs), can lead to learning disabilities and lower IQ scores.

Toxins in the home

The majority of homes now contain hundreds of chemicals. Chemical cleaning compounds and fabric protectors are two sources of chemicals that contaminate the household environment. We are told that these chemicals are safe as long as exposure to them is at or below the recommended level. But are they really safe?

Bruce Lanphear is an environmental health expert at Simon Fraser University in British Columbia. In a 2015 paper in *The Annual Review of Public Health*, he argues that when viewed in isolation, toxins may appear to be safe, but the cumulative effect of toxins on children's intellectual abilities has been underestimated.

The following is a list of chemicals that may occur in the food, water, or environment in your home. Since they affect the brain, they all have a detrimental effect on IQ. Parents should be aware of them and take measures to minimise the degree to which their children are exposed to them.

Arsenic: Exposure to arsenic impacts not only the brain, but almost every organ in the body. In 2014, in a review of the evidence of arsenic neurotoxicity children and adults, Tyler and Allan stated that arsenic toxicity is a worldwide health concern affecting several millions of people, who are exposed to it through drinking water. Arsenic's effect on IQ was also highlighted by researchers studying the effect on well water on the IQ of 272 children in Maine, US. They found that children whose drinking water contained 5μg/L or more arsenic had IQ scores 5-6 points lower than children whose drinking water contained less than 5μg/L.

Professor Andy Meharg of Queen's University Belfast expressed particular concern about the effect of arsenic on children and babies. He was quoted on the BBC website (February 2017), *"We know that low levels of arsenic impact immune development, they impact growth development, they impact IQ development."*

If you are concerned or curious about how much arsenic is in your water, you can write to your water authority and ask them for the arsenic content of your tap water. Alternatively, a search online for "arsenic test kit" will bring up many reasonably priced do-it-yourself test kits. The advantage of the home test kit is that you can also use it to test bottled water.

Rice is also a source of arsenic that affects millions of people because of its role as a staple of the global diet. Rice is prone to taking up more arsenic than other cereal foods and, because of this, it is a leading dietary source of inorganic arsenic — the most toxic type of arsenic. There are articles online that provide details about the brands of rice and rice products that are the worst offenders. Searching using the terms "arsenic in rice brand names" should return several articles to which you can refer.

Raab et al, *Journal of Environmental Monitoring*, (2009) recommend rinsing rice in clean water several times before cooking. After rinsing, the rice should be cooked in a large volume of water e.g. 6 cups of water for each cup of rice. The researchers found that this procedure can reduce the amount of inorganic arsenic in the cooked rice by as much as 45%.

In the UK, the Food Standards Agency (FSA) advises against giving toddlers and young children (1 – 4.5 years) rice drinks as a substitute for breast milk, infant formula, or cows' milk.

Bisphenol-A (BPA): BPA and its replacement bisphenol-S (BPS) are endocrine-disrupting chemicals. The United Nations Environment Program (UNEP) issued a report in February 2014 titled *State of the Science of Endocrine Disrupting Chemicals*. In the report stated, the authors elaborate on the extent to which BPA can disrupt all hormonal systems. Such a widescale disruption can lead to *"obesity, infertility or reduced fertility, learning and memory difficulties, adult-onset diabetes or cardiovascular disease, as well as a variety of other diseases."*

Bisphenol-A (BPA) is found in the liner of canned goods, numerous personal care and plastic products, plastic- and non-stick food containers, plastic wrapping materials, and water bottles.

You can reduce your exposure to BPA in the following ways:

- Use glass or steel water bottles and storage containers instead of plastic.
- Use fresh or frozen food in preference to canned foods.
- Avoid non-stick kitchen utensils.
- Always look for "non-toxic" on the label of products you buy. If in doubt, contact the manufacturer and ask them what the product is made from.
- Do not heat up toxic plastics in microwave or traditional ovens.

Flame Retardants: Flame retardants are chemicals that are used to treat textiles, plastics, and other flammable materials to reduce the effect of fires on people, property, and the environment.

A 2013 study investigating the effect of exposure to flame retardants studied 309 pregnant women. Blood analysis showed that a specific class of retardant, polybrominated diphenyl ethers (PBDEs), was clearly present in the blood. The researchers tracked the children of these women with high levels of PBDEs through the first five years of their lives and found that the children showed increased rates of hyperactivity between ages two to five and cognition deficits at the age of 5. When PBDE levels increase from 10 parts per billion (PPB) to 100 ppb, a child's IQ decreases by 5 points. A similar effect is seen when children are exposed to organophosphate pesticides early in life.

Given that reducing the likelihood of fires by putting obstacles such as flame retardants in the way is a good thing to do, how can parents reconcile the advantages of chemical fire retardants with their negative impact on IQ? The California Childcare Health Program has the following useful suggestions in their factsheet *Minimizing Exposure to Toxic Flame-Retardants*:

- Fire-retardant chemicals stick to the hands, so wash hands frequently.

- Try to source furniture of a type that is less likely to contain fire retardants, for example, wooden furniture or furniture filled with down, wool, cotton, or polyester.

- Check with the manufacturer of the furniture you intend buy to see whether the furniture is sprayed with PBDE containing chemicals. If you are buying upholstered furniture, look for furniture that has the foam firmly encased inside a thick outer cover so that there's less leakage of toxic chemicals.

- Buy a vacuum cleaner with a High Efficiency Particulate Air (HEPA) filter.

- Carpets and curtains are likely to be treated with flame retardants. Laminate and vinyl flooring are also known to be toxic. Non-toxic flooring alternatives include ceramic tiles, hardwood flooring, linoleum, and bare floorboards. If you choose to have carpets, use rugs that can be cleaned outside.

Strides are being made to develop non-toxic flame retardants (*ScienceDaily*, Jul 2013). A search online for "natural fire retardants" will yield a whole host of information about non-toxic fire retardants including homemade recipes that can be used as replacements for toxic flame retardants.

Fluoride: Fluoride has long been touted as an effective and safe way of improving dental health, but research is emerging that shows it is far from safe. *The Lancet* (February 2014) published a study by Dr Philippe Grandjean, MD and Dr Philip J Landrigan, MD that classified fluoride as a neurotoxin alongside 11 other neurotoxins.

A 2012 paper written by researchers from Harvard School of Public Health (HSPH) and China Medical University in Shenyang titled *Developmental Fluoride Neurotoxicity: A Systematic Review and Meta-Analysis* reviewed 27 published studies on the effect of fluoride. The researchers concluded that children in high-fluoride areas had an IQ score 7 points lower than those who lived in low fluoride areas.

Dr Yan Lu, Department of Environmental Health, Tianjin Medical University, Tianjin, China conducted a study to measure the effect of water with a high fluoride level on the intelligence of children. In the study, the IQ of 118 children aged 10-12 was compared. Sixty children were from an area where there was high fluoride level in the drinking water. The remainder of the children were from a low-fluoride area. The results showed that the IQ of the children in the high-fluoride area was nearly 11 points lower than the children in the low-fluoride region.

Reduce the amount of fluoride that your children ingest by only allowing them to drink tap or bottled water that has not been artificially fluoridated. If you live in an area where tap water is fluoridated and you don't want to use bottled water, you could install a water filter that removes fluoride.

Lead: The toxic effects of lead are well documented. A study was published in the *New England Journal of Medicine* in which the levels of lead in the blood of 172 children ranging from six months to 5 years was measured. Researchers tested the children's IQ at ages 3 and 5. They found that the children with blood levels of lead that had increased from one microgram per decilitre to ten micrograms per decilitre (the limit under CDC's safety guidelines) experienced an IQ drop of 7.4 points.

Alan Kaufman published an article in the *Archives of Clinical Neuropsychology* titled *Do low levels of lead produce IQ loss in children? A careful examination of the literature* (2001). In this article, Kaufman presents the findings of his exhaustive analysis of 26 well-controlled studies on the impact of lead on children's intelligence. Although he found many shortcomings in the best lead-IQ studies, many of the investigators have reported an IQ loss of around 3 points due to lead.

Lead exposure in young children can result in a permanent loss of IQ as well as a decrease in attention span and demonstration of anti-social behaviours.

Tamara Rubin helped form Lead Safe America. Visit their site (http://leadsafeamerica.org/) to learn everything you need to know about lead poisoning, from testing to what products to avoid, to help on how to help your family avoid lead in your home.

Manganese: Manganese (Mn) is used widely in the production of steel, aluminium alloys, batteries, and fertilizers and it is also added to unleaded gasoline. It plays a key role in brain growth and development, but excessive amounts can result in neurotoxicity. Manganese appears in water, soil, and the air as a result of industrial emissions and other causes. Another source is soy and rice beverages.

The effect of manganese on IQ was the subject of a study titled *Manganese Exposure and Neurocognitive Outcomes in Rural School-Age Children* (October 2015). The researchers found that children with blood levels of Mn greater than 11.2 micrograms/L had an IQ score that was 3.51 points lower than children with an Mn blood level between 8.2 and 11.2 micrograms/L. Another study, published in *Environmental Health Perspectives* (2010), reported a drop in IQ of up to 6 points in a group of 362 Quebec children who consumed tap water that contained manganese.

You can buy test kits online to see whether your water is contaminated with manganese. If the water is contaminated, filters are available that can remove up to 100% of manganese.

Cockell et al, Journal of the American College of Nutrition, (2004) recommend that soy beverages and rice beverages should not be fed to infants.

Mercury: Methylmercury, a form of mercury is listed in *The Lancet* as a neurotoxin.

A May 2005 article in *Environment Health Perspectives* titled *Public Health and Economic Consequences of Methyl Mercury Toxicity to the Developing Brain* cites three recent, large-scale studies that have examined children who experienced methyl mercury exposures whilst in the womb. The first of these studies, a group in New Zealand, found a 3-point decrease in IQ in a population that regularly consumed methylmercury-contaminated fish during pregnancy.

Another study in the same journal (August 2015) examined the

Relation of Prenatal Methylmercury Exposure from Environmental Sources to Childhood IQ. The results showed that prenatal mercury was associated with poorer performance. The IQ scores of the more heavily exposed children were 4.8 points lower on average than the less heavily exposed children.

Reduce exposure to mercury by having mercury tooth fillings replaced with non-toxic filling, and sourcing fish and produce that are mercury-free. Energy efficient lighting can contain mercury so dispose of it very carefully, taking great care not to break the bulbs.

Mercury is a widely-studied neurotoxin that, if ingested during pregnancy, has been shown to reduce the IQ of the developing baby.

Mould: Mould has been linked to respiratory infections, allergies, and asthma. A study assessing the exposure to indoor mould and its effect on the cognitive function of 6-year-old children was published in *Physiology Behavior* (October 2011).

The study was based on the six-year follow-up of 277 babies born in Krakow, Poland. All the women included in the study were, at the time of pregnancy, non-smokers and free of chronic diseases such as diabetes and hypertension. The researchers found that children who lived for longer periods in mould-contaminated dwellings scored about 10 points lower than those with no exposure to mould.

Organophosphate (OP) pesticides: A joint research project across several universities in the U.S. and Canada looked at the effect of exposure to OP pesticides during and after pregnancy on the cognitive abilities children of school age. The results showed that the concentration of Diammonium Phosphate (DAP) found in the urine of pregnant women was associated with poorer intellectual development in 7-year-old children. The children of mothers with the highest DAP concentrations in their urine had, on average, an IQ that was 7 points lower than the children of mothers with the lowest DAP concentrations.

Phthalates: There are two types of phthalates that are commonly found in homes. They are di-n-butyl phthalate (DnBP) and di-isobutyl phthalate (DiBP). Both are found in a wide variety of consumer products, from dryer sheets to vinyl fabrics and personal care products such as lipstick, hairspray, nail polish, and even some soaps.

A study published in the December 2014 issue of *PLOS ONE* reported the effects of exposure to phthalates during pregnancy and the subsequent effect on IQ of children. Researchers from Columbia University's Mailman School of Public Health did a follow up on 328 inner-city mothers. They found that, at the age of 7, children exposed to high levels of two common chemicals found in the home (DnBP and DiBP) during pregnancy had an IQ score, on average, more than 6 points lower than children who had been exposed at lower levels.

Alternative non-toxic versions of many of the products that contain phthalates are now readily available. They may be slightly more expensive, but the extra cost would be money well spent.

PVC: Polyvinyl chloride (PVC) is widely used in the construction industry, packaging product, and many other domestic and other consumer products. In its "raw" state, PVC is a highly unstable and so it requires various additives to prevent it breaking down. Of the chemicals added to PVC to stabilise and modify its physical and mechanical properties, some are known to be toxic. Nonetheless, they continue to be used for economic reasons and because there is no legislative mechanism or incentive to control their use. **Lead compounds**, for example, are still routinely used in many PVC products, particularly those used in the construction industry, and lead is detrimental to IQ.

How do I find out how many toxins are in my child's body?

Knowing the levels of toxic chemicals in your child's body is useful to find out the source of and severity of exposure to environmental toxins. Armed with this information, you will be able to take focused action to prioritise the removal of any toxins that are discovered during testing.

Accurately testing for toxins is not an easy process and full testing involves analysis of hair, urine, and faeces using sophisticated scientific instruments. If you are interested, then you can search online for a testing laboratory or consult your doctor for guidance.

KEEP YOUR CHILDREN AWAY FROM TOXINS

Most of the information outlined in this chapter focuses on the negative effect of toxins on IQ, however, the negative impact of toxins extends way beyond a low IQ. The debilitating effects on health and wellbeing are too serious to ignore and for this reason, parents must take every precaution to protect their children and the whole family from toxins:

- Some tap water is artificially fluoridated. Ask your water supplier if your water supply is fluoridated. If it is, then you may want to consider installing a water filter to remove fluoride from your drinking supply or use only drinking bottled water.

- Fluoride occurs naturally in many bottled waters, but some bottled waters are artificially fluoridated. The ones that are artificially fluoridated should be labelled, so check the label if you want to avoid these brands. Alternatively, you can check on www.bottledwater.org.

- To reduce the arsenic content in rice, cook rice in a 6:1 ratio of water to rice and discard the excess water after.

- Have silver-mercury fillings removed by a specialist dentist.

- Search online for "toxin-free fish" or "toxin-free seafood" to find out how to identify and source toxin-free seafood.

- Chemical flame retardants make environments safer but currently, most are toxic. Alternative non-toxic versions are being researched and developed. In the meantime, follow some of the guidelines listed earlier in the chapter.

- Check for and eliminate sources of lead in your house.

- Eat fresh organic produce that is free of brain-damaging pesticides.

- Where possible, avoid using plastic products to avoid BPA contamination.

- Use only natural household cleaners such as vinegar, lemon, and bicarbonate of soda. Search online for "natural cleaner recipes".

- Avoid using chemical-based pest control products.

- Check the label of everything you buy for baby to make sure that they are phthalate-free.

- Avoid buying plastic products that contain PVC or phthalates. There may be information on the label, but if there isn't, you can contact the manufacturers for more information.

- Avoid eating food stored or microwaved in PVC plastic containers.

- Keep indoor rooms well-ventilated to avoid the development and build-up of mould. There are humidifiers that literally suck mould out of the air. You may want to invest in one.

- Buy plants that purify the air in your home. You can discover what is available through on online search or ask at your local gardening centre.

- You may want to consider having a toxicity analysis for your children (and yourself).

16

Physical Exercise

"To keep the body in good health is a duty, otherwise we shall not be able to keep our mind strong and clear."

Buddha

Almost everyone appreciates that exercise is good for the body. The benefits of exercise include better health, better mood, more energy, and weight control. In addition to these physical benefits, numerous studies have linked exercise to better brain health. For example, one recent BBC online article cited a German study where children who walked to school tended to display better concentration and get better test results than those who were driven to school. In this chapter, we'll examine how IQ can be improved through exercise.

"We all know that exercise makes us feel better, but most of us have no idea why," says Harvard Medical School Psychiatry Professor John J. Ratey, MD. *"We assume it's because we're burning off stress or reducing muscle tension, or boosting endorphins,"* he explains. *"But the real reason we feel so good when we get our blood pumping is that it makes the brain function at its best … I often tell my patients that the point of exercise is to build and condition the brain."*

Children make themselves smarter when they take part in sports and other physical activity. Exercise has "a more long-lasting effect on brains that are still developing," says Phil Tomporowski, Exercise Science Professor at the University of Georgia.

Exercise benefits intelligence

There is a huge amount of research demonstrating that exercise benefits intelligence, some of which we'll look at now.

A review of the research literature pertaining to physical activity, fitness, cognitive function, and academic achievement in children was published in the *Journal of American College of Sports Medicine, (2016)*. The authors concluded that physical activity positively affects brain structure and function as well as cognition.

In *Health Psychology* (January 2011), Catherine Davis et al showed that 40 minutes of exercise a day for 3 months improved intelligence scores of overweight children by nearly 4 points.

Hillman et al (2014) studied more than 220 school children and found that children who engaged in 60 minutes of aerobic activities daily after school performed better on tests relating to focus and cognitive flexibility, that is, the ability to switch between tasks while maintaining speed and accuracy. In another study of 20 children, Hillman et al (2009) found that 20 minutes of walking on a treadmill increased children's subsequent performance on tests of reading comprehension.

Swedish researchers analysed the results of both physical and IQ tests of 1.2 million Swedish men and found a clear link between good physical fitness and better IQ test results. The strongest were in the areas of logical thinking and verbal comprehension.

Physical exercise can be used to increase both fitness and strength. However, Michael Nilsson, professor at the Sahlgrenska Academy, stated that fitness, not strength, plays a role in increasing IQ. He states, "Being fit means that you also have good heart and lung capacity and that your brain gets plenty of oxygen". Therefore, increased fitness should be the end goal of any physical exercise program targeted at improving your child's IQ.

A strategy for better exam performance

Several studies show that physical exercise before a test helps children get better results.

The Trends in International Mathematics and Science Study (TIMSS) test is an international benchmarking test that measures students' performance. In 1999, the TIMSS test was given to 230,000 students from thirty-eight countries. There were 59,000 participants from the United States, and one of the districts that participated was Naperville.

To the surprise of many, Naperville's students were ranked number one in Science and sixth in Maths — behind only Singapore, Korea, Taiwan, Hong Kong and Japan. Generally, U.S. students placed eighteenth in science and nineteenth in math. Districts from Jersey City and Miami coming last in science and math, respectively.

What led to Naperville's remarkable success? The district attributed the success to a new physical education class. Students who took the class directly one hour before the test had improved reading and maths scores of 20%. Following the TIMSS results, guidance counsellors at the school advised all students to arrange their schedule such that their most difficult subjects are immediately after gym.

Howie et al (2005) conducted a study where 96 children who exercised 10-20 minutes prior to a maths test outperformed children in the inactive control group.

Similarly, Winter et al (2007), in the journal *Neurobiology or Learning and Memory,* reported that vocabulary learning was 20% faster after intense physical exercise.

The lesson here is that children who are already fit and active could benefit from a short burst of physical training before an examination or test.

EXERCISE INCREASES INTELLIGENCE

Exercise should be one of the cornerstones of a parent's strategy to increase their child's IQ. To reap the benefits of exercise, a child does not need to follow a specific regimen unless that's what they want to do. A game of football, a ride on the bike or other bursts of activity will work wonders.

Here are some examples of how you can get the ball rolling:

- Ensure that your children take part in physical activities from an early age. The sooner they start, the sooner it will become a part of their psyche — make fitness a priority in your home.

- Be a role model. Kids whose parents are active will also be inclined to be active. Go for walks, run, bike or take part in sports. If you make it fun, your kids will want to follow in your footsteps.

- Every weekend, make it a point to do something active with your children such as swimming, going to the park, or playing football.

- Let your child choose activities that they like. The easiest way to get children interested in exercise at a young age is to keep it fun.

- Most physical activities can count as exercise. Get your children involved in dancing, hiking in the woods, swimming, cycling, jogging, soccer, or taking the dog out for a walk. There's even video games available that require players to move around quite vigorously — such as tennis and dance games.

- As a family, enrol in a fun run or a walk for charity.

- Physical activity before tests has been proven to increase test scores.

17

The Importance of Sleep

"Your life is a reflection of how you sleep, and how you sleep is a reflection of your life."

Dr. Rafael Pelayo, Clinical Professor,
Stanford Center for Sleep Sciences and Medicine

Sleep is a key component of a healthy life. During sleep, the mind and body rejuvenate, the brain processes new memories, and our body releases hormones to regulate growth and appetite. If sleep is cut short, then we wake up less prepared, less able to focus and concentrate, and with a compromised ability to make decisions and perform at work and school. The lack of adequate, good-quality sleep has been shown to hinder cognitive functioning in children and adversely affect behaviour, health, and IQ.

How sleep affects IQ

The *Journal of Pediatrics* (2012) published results from a study of 1,385 children of approximately 6 years of age who had a range of sleep problems. These problems were being unwilling to sleep alone, talking in their sleep, having difficulty maintaining sleep, sleep resistance, sleeping less, nightmares, fatigue, and lack of energy. The researchers discovered that compared to children who had no sleep problems at all, children with fatigue had scores 3-6 points lower on IQ and those with other sleep problems scored 2-3 points lower on IQ.

Another study published in *Child Development* (2003), investigated how reducing and increasing the amount of sleep by 30 minutes affected the performance of 77 fourth and sixth-graders. Half of the group were given an extra 30 minutes of sleep while the other half had their sleep period reduced by 30 minutes. The authors concluded that the effect of even 30 minutes of sleep deprivation has significant implications for learning and school performance. Dr Avi Sadeh, lead author has indicated that the loss of one hour of sleep can make a 6th grader perform at the level of a 4th grader.

Computers, video games, smartphones, tablets, and TVs are ubiquitous. Multiple devices can often be found in almost every room of every home, certainly in developed nations at least. Given that multiple screens may be flashing away during most evenings, the question arises whether there is any impact of these devices on children and their sleep. A paper published in *JAMA Pedriatrics* (2016) looked at 20 peer reviewed studies to answer this question. The results of the analysis concluded that bedtime use of a media device was significantly associated with inadequate sleep quantity, poor sleep quality, and excessive daytime sleepiness.

Foley et al (2017) monitored how much time children and teens spent watching TV and playing video games in the 90 minutes before their bedtimes. They found that the children who watched the most TV and played the most video games in the 90 minutes before bed took longer to fall asleep compared to children who watched less TV or played video games for a shorter time, or not at all. Based on this evidence, parents should cut off device access well before bedtime - preferably several hours before.

Some parents allow young children to stay up late on Fridays and Saturdays. According to Dr Monique LeBourgeois, a researcher of kindergartner sleep patterns, the cost of this is a 7-point drop on a test to measure school-readiness. The results, presented at the conference *Sleep 2006*, indicated that this drop is seen even though the children are not sleep deprived.

A lack of sleep also contributes to a poorer vocabulary, a factor that affects IQ. Dr Paul Suratt of the University of Virginia studied how sleep problems affected the vocabulary-test scores of elementary-school students. His findings, published in the journal *Pediatrics* (2006), demonstrated that as a result of sleep problems, vocabulary test scores dropped by 7 points. Dr Suratt explains that *"vocabulary scores are known to be the best single predictor of a child's IQ and the strongest predictor of academic success"*.

The book *Nurture Shock (2009)* reported the results of a survey of more than 7,000 high schoolers in Minnesota on their sleep habits and grades. The researcher, Dr Kyla Wahlstrom, discovered that teens who achieved A grades averaged about fifteen minutes of extra sleep compared to students who achieved Bs. Likewise, the students who attained Bs averaged eleven more minutes of sleep than students who received a C. C students slept ten more minutes than the Ds.

Through his research, Professor Joseph Buckhalt has discovered that poor sleep affects the performance of children with higher intelligence to a greater degree than those with lower intelligence (*Psychology Today, 2015*). In the same article, he discusses evidence that children living in poverty have lower school performance and poorer sleep than middle and upper-class children. Based on this, he suggests that ensuring improved sleep for lower class children may lead to better school performance, and that children with higher IQs may have even more to gain by improving sleep.

These dips in IQ appear to be temporary if the sleep deficit is reversed. However, in the case of children, even a temporary deficit can have severe implications on performance at school, especially just before and during tests.

What constitutes healthy sleep?

The National Sleep Foundation lists the following components of healthy sleep:

- Falling asleep within minutes of lying down.
- Sleep duration is age-appropriate.
- Sleep is continuous and undisturbed.
- Upon awakening, there is a feeling of being refreshed.
- During the day, there is a feeling of being productive and alert (allowing the occasional dip such as after a meal).
- There are no indications of restlessness, snoring, pauses in breathing, nightmares, or other abnormal behaviours.

How much sleep do children need?

According the National Sleep Foundation, sleep needs vary according to age:

Category	Age	Hours of Sleep Required
New-borns	1-2 months	10.5-18 hours
Infants	3-11 months	9-12 hours at night plus 1-4 naps during the day
Toddlers	1-3 years	12-14 hours
Pre-schoolers	3-5 years	11-13 hours
School-aged children	5-12 years	10-11 hours
Teens	11-17 years	8.5-9.25 hours

Touchette et al (2007) followed the sleep patterns of 1,492 children aged from 5 months to 6 years. They found that a consistent reduction of 1 hour of sleep at night during early childhood led to a threefold increase in the risk of low performance on IQ tests. In their conclusion, they highlighted the importance of children having at least 10 hours of sleep per night throughout early childhood.

For younger children, the more sleep, the better!

ENSURE CHILDREN GET ADEQUATE HIGH QUALITY SLEEP

Studies indicate that adequate sleep is required for optimum brain functioning and overall health. If children don't get sufficient high-quality sleep, their IQ and performance at school will suffer.

- Ensure that your children get enough sleep for their age and that the environment is comfortable, quiet, and conducive to high-quality sleep. If your child complains of being tired even though you feel that the environment is adequate, try setting earlier bedtimes or consult your doctor, who may be able to offer advice or point you towards a sleep clinic.

- Too much activity before bedtime can contribute to difficulty falling asleep. Help your child to relax hours before bedtime and stop them overstimulating their brains with TV, video games, and other electronic devices during the 90 minutes before bedtime.

- As far as possible, keep to a regular sleep schedule. Weekend late passes impact on a child's performance after the weekend.

- More sleep is better than less. Reducing sleep by even 15 minutes has been shown to reduce academic achievement.

18

Breath Power

"Regulate the breathing, and thereby control the mind."

– B.K.S. Iyengar, founder of Iyengar Yoga

Babies and young children naturally breathe correctly — it's second nature. But over time, our breathing habits change. We often start to constrict our abdomens and breathe mainly into our chests. This restricts our oxygen intake and can lead to problems such as anxiety, poor concentration, and even a drop in IQ. Moving from poor breathing habits to good breathing habits can lead to a profound improvement in both health and intelligence.

According to Dr Win Wenger, a pioneer in the fields of mind and brain development, the breath paces and punctuates attention and awareness. That is, as soon as we start to pay attention to something, we hold our breath. Then, when we are ready to move our attention to the next thing, we take another breath and so on. If our breathing pattern breaks our attention before we finish reading a sentence, it can be difficult to make sense of and extract meaning from that sentence. We may have to bring our attention back to the sentence and refocus on it until the meaning of the sentence becomes clear in our mind.

What this means in simple terms is that, if the duration of our breaths is shorter than the sentences that we read, we may continually have to go back to re-focus on those sentences to make sense of them. As a result, there will be problems with reading comprehension.

Dr Wenger asserts that *"the normal span of your breath is critical to how well your mental faculties can function"*. He goes on to say that, whilst many situations have the *potential* to induce, short attention-span, hyperactivity and reading problems, being short of breath virtually guarantees their occurrence.

How do you recognise poor breathing?

It is a good idea to check your child's breathing and if needed, take corrective action. The following table lists the various types of **poor breathing habits** and how to recognise them.

Bad Breathing Habit	Symptom
Mouth breathing	Mouth breathing is easily identified. This is the type of breathing that happens when you have a cold and your nose is blocked.
Shallow breathing	Lie on your back and place one hand on your lower ribs. When you breathe, if you can't feel your lower ribs moving along with your belly, then your breathing is too shallow.
Upper chest breathing	When you take a breath and the chest moves before the abdomen, that is upper chest breathing.
Over breathing	Over breathing happens when your inhalation goes on for longer than your exhalation. In correct breathing, your inhalation should take slightly longer than your exhalation.
Reverse breathing	During normal breathing, the diaphragm goes down during inhalation. In reverse breathing, the diaphragm drops down instead of coming up.
Breath retention	Breath retention is very common. If you observe yourself, you'll be surprised how often you unconsciously hold your breath during your daily activities.

All these modes of breathing can have an impact on the amount of oxygen going to the brain and some, such as mouth breathing, can be the cause of life-threatening conditions.

The effects of mouth breathing and IQ

In the study, *An Evaluation on the Relation between Chronic Mouth*

Breathing and Childrens IQ, researchers compared the IQs of 60 otherwise healthy children aged 6-12 years who were diagnosed as mouth breathers with 60 children who were not. They found that mouth-breathing children had IQs almost 3 points lower than the control group.

A 2015 study published in the *Sao Paulo Medical Journal* looked at deficits in working memory, reading comprehension, and arithmetic skills of 42 children who were mouth breathers. The study reported that compared to normal breathers, the mouth breathers had poorer academic achievement and cognitive skills than the control children. The researchers stated that in general, mouth breathing impairs children's overall health by causing daytime tiredness and loss of attention.

Snoring and sleep apnea

Obstructive sleep apnea (OSA) is a disorder in which a person pauses their breathing during sleep. The pauses can last from a few seconds to minutes. Several studies have established the negative impact of OSA on IQ. Blunden et al (2000) reported that children who snore had impaired attention and lower memory and intelligence scores. Kennedy et al (2004) found that children who snored had a mean global IQ score of 97 compared to non-snorers who scored 110.

A 2006 study investigating the link between childhood sleep apnea and IQ found that OSA in children can lead to brain cell damage and lowered IQ. The researchers found that the mean IQ score of children with sleep apnea was 85 compared to 101 for healthy children. Lead author Ann Halbower stated that untreated, the IQ-damaging effects of sleep apnea could become permanent. The sooner the condition is diagnosed and treated, the lower the risk of permanent damage.

As well as a decrease in IQ, OSA is linked to many other serious health issues. Clues that your child may be at risk from OSA include the following:

- Snoring, often with snorts, pauses or gasps.
- Loud, heavy breathing during sleep.
- Extremely restless sleep.

- Unusual sleeping positions, for example, with the rear end up in the air and head tilted.

If you suspect that your child has sleep apnea, you should seek medical advice as soon as possible.

Just as poor breathing can lead to problems such as anxiety, anxiety can be the cause of poor breathing — it's a two-way street. If your child breathes noisily or irregularly, there may be underlying health issues. You should seek medical advice to investigate this possibility.

Correct breathing

Proper breathing is breathing through the nose and largely involves the diaphragm, the large sheet-like muscle that lies at the bottom of the chest cavity. 70 – 80% of the inhaling should be done using the diaphragm. The remaining 20-30% involves muscles in the abdomen, chest, neck, and shoulders. There are many articles and videos online that demonstrate correct breathing techniques.

Nose breathing combined with deep breathing is a good lifetime habit and there is evidence that it helps to improve your child's performance. *The Lancet* (1998) published a study listed some of the benefits of nasal breathing: increased blood oxygen, and carbon dioxide levels, better circulation, a lower breathing rate, and improved overall lung volumes. Anything that increase blood oxygen is a boost to the brain.

Further benefits of nasal breathing are listed in the *International Journal of Neuroscience* (1993) where it is stated that *"increased airflow through the right nostril is correlated to increased left brain activity and enhanced verbal performance, whereas increased airflow through the left nostril is associated with increased right brain activity and enhanced spatial performance."*

Generally, nose breathing works the diaphragm harder, causing the lungs to pull in more air. It is a simple way and quick way to give brain function a boost.

An exceptional result

A dramatic and possibly unique illustration of how deep breathing can improve IQ can be found in a 2000 CIA report *Experimental Research in the Application of Qigong (Deep Breathing) Exercises to Restore Intelligence for Mentally Handicapped Children*. The research was undertaken by The Somatic Science Research Office of Yunnan University's Physics department. In the paper, they discussed the case of a 12-year old girl with an initial verbal IQ of 40 that increased to 70 after this Qigong breathing therapy. The study authors concluded that *"Practical results prove that Qigong intelligence recovery therapy can alter the state of low functional ability of the cerebral brain cells of mentally handicapped children. It only requires enough time for such Qigong intelligence restoration therapy, and the intelligence of feeble-minded children can be raised even to normal levels."*

Correct breathing involves breathing deeply through the nose. Deep breathing infuses oxygen into the blood and therefore the brain, and enhances its functioning. By breathing incorrectly, your child may be robbing the brain of the oxygen it needs to work at peak efficiency.

A possible caveat to deep breathing

A 2008 study published in the *American Journal of Epidemiology* found that breathing dirty air may lower a child's IQ. The study looked at 202 Boston children aged 8 to 11 who lived in neighbourhoods with heavy traffic pollution. They found that heavy exposure to black carbon was linked to a 3.4 point drop in IQ. They also scored worse on other tests of intelligence and memory compared to children who breathe cleaner air.

Deep breathing is a desirable habit and should be encouraged. However, parents should be conscious of environmental conditions such as mould and pollution that may undermine any potential IQ gains. The nose has its own defence against pollution — hairs, but they can only trap some pollutants. In areas with high levels of pollution, additional measures should be taken. Inside, house plants and filters can help to keep the air clean. Outside, children can wear masks such as the ones cyclists wear.

CORRECT BREATHING INCREASES IQ

Every cell in our body needs oxygen to function effectively. Good breathing maximises oxygen intake, which provides the oxygen that the brain needs to perform optimally. Poor breathing deprives your child's body of the oxygen that it needs to fully feed the developing brain.

Here are some things you can do to help your child improve their breathing:

- Train your children to become aware of how they breathe so that they can catch themselves out when they are breathing incorrectly.

- Teach them to breathe deeply by practising diaphragmatic breathing.

- Enrol them in singing lessons. Correct singing requires diaphragmatic breathing, and one of the first things that vocal coaches teach is correct breathing.

- Encourage your child to breathe through their nose. If they are a chronic mouth breather, take them to the doctor or the dentist. A doctor or dentist trained in airway management will be able to assess the reason why your child breathes through their mouth.

- If you live in an area with a lot of air pollution, take measures to minimise the impact of the pollution on your children, such as:

  - Don't let children go outdoors during periods of heavy pollution such as the rush hour unless it's absolutely necessary.

  - Encourage them to breathe through their nose. The nose has hairs that act as a filter and trap macro pollutants.

- To enhance the effect of nose hairs when your children are outside, consider making them wear masks — such as the ones that cyclists wear. That is, if you can find a type that are comfortable and safe for children.
- Buy air purifiers for the house.
- Increase greenery in and around the house.
- If the pollution is particularly bad, consider moving to a cleaner area.

19

Health Issues That Impact IQ

"When health is absent, wisdom cannot reveal itself, art cannot manifest, strength cannot fight, wealth becomes useless, and intelligence cannot be applied."

Herophilus, Greek physician and the world's first anatomist

There are a number of health conditions that impact IQ. Whilst IQ is probably the last thing on your mind when your child is ill, there is value in being aware of these conditions for two reasons. Firstly, you can take measures in your home, other environments, and your lifestyle to reduce the likelihood of your child falling victim to these diseases. Secondly, your child's alertness or intellectual abilities can act as a barometer — a tool to gauge your child's health. For example, if your child's alertness and mental acuity are degrading and there is no obvious cause, it could be a sign of an underlying illness that may need medical attention.

Secondary smoke: Second-hand smoke can decrease a child's IQ. A study of 4,399 children published in *Environmental Health Perspectives (2005)* reported drops in IQ scores of between 2 to 5 points depending upon the levels of exposure to secondary smoke. Even exposure to a small amount of cigarette smoke can lower cognitive abilities. One parent smoking less than a pack a day could reduce the IQ scores of the child by an average of 2 points.

Stress: Childhood stress comes in many forms, such as verbal abuse, violence and arguing in the home, bullying, corporal punishment, negative news on the TV, and even overhearing parents talking about their own problems.

Many parents are noticing that the ever-increasing barrage of tests in school and homework is causing children to feel overwhelmed. In one recent widely reported case, a mother wrote to her daughter's school saying how her daughter is *"very stressed and is starting to have physical symptoms such as chest pain and waking up at 4am worrying about her school workload"*.

Bernard Brown and Lilian Rosenbaum of Georgetown University created a stress index using a sample of 4,000 children aged 7. They found that children who are under emotional or physical stress show a drop in IQ scores from 104 with no stress to 91 under high stress.

How can parents help children who are feeling stressed? The first thing is to be there for your child. Next, listen attentively and calmly. Once you understand the issue, you can work with your child to come up with solutions. There is no one solution that fits all cases, but sometimes simple actions such as taking time out to play, exercise, listen to relaxing music, or doing meditation can being to calm a troubled mind. Stress hormones profoundly affect the brain so if the situation persists, parents should seek a drug-free solution through a qualified practitioner.

Diabetes: According to the International Diabetes Federation, in 2015 there were 415 million people with diabetes, and this is projected to increase to 642 million by 2040.

There are two principle types of diabetes. In Type 1, there is a lack of insulin production and in Type 2, insulin is produced but used ineffectively by the body. Type 2 often results from excess body weight and lack of physical activity. Type 2 used to occur nearly entirely among adults, but now occurs in children too (*WHO 2016 Global Report on Diabetes*).

Children and Young People Diabetes (2015), published by Healthy London Partnership, Diabetes UK, and South East Coast and London Diabetes Partnership Board, listed the following intelligence related observations based on scientific research:

- Continued and chronic exposure to the effects of diabetes is related to poorer learning and school achievement, especially in reading and spelling. Children whose diabetes developed later in childhood or during adolescence also had poorer scores on tests of vocabulary and general knowledge.

- Severe episodes of low blood glucose levels (hypoglycaemia) lead to lower verbal and full scale IQ at six years after diagnosis.

- The age at which hypoglycaemic events (such as seizures) begin rather than the age of onset of the illness is related to reduced verbal and visual delayed recall and spatial intelligence.

- Hyperglycaemia (elevated blood sugar levels) has a detrimental effect on information processing speed, verbal intelligence, the ability to maintain attention and spatial intelligence. Memory is also negatively affected.

- Puberty can lead to complications of diabetes due to hormonal changes.

- Children with diabetes have been reported to achieve average and high average IQ scores, though the group average was still three to seven points lower than the control group.

To help reduce the risk of your child getting diabetes:

- Ensure your child eats healthily and regularly takes part in physical activities.

- Be aware of the key symptoms of diabetes: increased thirst and hunger, frequent urination, weight loss or gain for no obvious cause, blurred vision, nausea, and wounds that heal slowly.

- If there is a family history of diabetes, be extra vigilant because the risk of your child developing diabetes may be heightened – take them for regular medical checks.

Toxoplasmosis: Toxoplasmosis is a parasitic infection that is important for women who are pregnant or intending to become pregnant to be aware of. If, during pregnancy, the infection spreads to baby, it could result in an IQ drop of 17 points as highlighted in the *Iranian Journal of Parasitology* (2012). Even worse, infection may lead to a miscarriage or stillbirth.

The parasite is found in the faeces of infected cats and in infected meat and is extremely common, occurring as it does in more than 50% of the population in Central and Southern Europe, Africa, South America, and Asia. According to the American Pregnancy

Association, 1 out 1,000-8,000 babies born in the U.S. are born with toxoplasmosis. Despite its prevalence, toxoplasmosis often goes unreported. This is largely because there may be no symptoms. Where there are symptoms, however, these could include fatigue, fever, and swollen lymph nodes.

There are a lot of pet cats in the world. The RSPCA reports that there are over 7.2 million pet cats in the UK. In the U.S., the number is greater with more pet cats than pet dogs: 75 million cats vs. nearly 70 million dogs. Throughout the world cats appear to be the most popular pet.

If you are exposed to or have cats or anyone in your family consumes minimally cooked or raw meat, it would be worthwhile paying to have a blood test to check for parasites. A blood test will reveal whether the toxoplasmosis parasite is present in the body.

The UK National Health Service (http://www.nhs.uk) lists a number of measures to reduce the risk of being infected by this parasite. They are:

- Always wash your hands before and after handling food — especially raw meat.
- Thoroughly wash all kitchenware after preparing raw meat.
- Wash fruit and vegetables before eating them — this includes pre-prepared salads and pre-washed vegetables.
- Do not drink unpasteurised goats milk and do not eat any products made from unpasteurized goats milk.
- Wear gloves when changing litter trays. Pregnant women should not change litter trays.
- If your child has a sandpit, keep it covered so cats cannot defecate there.
- Feed your cat canned meat instead of raw meat, which may be infected.

Malaria: Malaria is a parasitic infection that is both preventable and curable. However, even if the malaria is cured, there is a post-malaria cognitive impairment that is often overlooked. This 'hidden' burden of malaria as it is termed by Fernando et al in the *Malaria Journal* (2010), could "have a long-lasting effect on patients' lives by preventing them from achieving their full potential".

According to the *World Malaria Report 2015*, there were 214 million cases of malaria globally in 2015. In the journal *Nature* (2015), the impact of malaria on IQ and cognition was quantified as follows:

- Cerebral malaria affects cognition, working memory, speech and language, attention, visual spatial skills, and receptive and expressive language.
- After one year of the episode, infected children exhibit a 13-point drop in IQ compared to non-affected children. Approximately 26% of children demonstrate impairment two years after.
- Acute malarial anaemia leads to the equivalent of an 11-point drop in IQ compared to malaria free children.

During diagnosis, Fernando et al state that *"attacks of cerebral malaria, coma, seizures and hypoglycaemia during an acute attack must be actively looked for and avoided to prevent later cognitive impairment."*

What can parents do to prevent their child getting malaria and to minimise the risk of there being any long-term consequences for IQ? The UK's National Health Service (NHS) recommends the following ABCD approach:

- **A**wareness of risk – check before travelling to see whether your destination is in a malaria zone.
- **B**ite prevention – take precautions to avoid bites. Use insect repellent, cover arms and legs, and use mosquito nets.
- **C**heck whether you need to take anti-malaria tablets and if you do, ensure you complete the course.
- **D**iagnosis – seek immediate medical advice if you have malaria symptoms.

Bacterial meningitis: Meningitis is an illness that most parents are aware of. It is contagious and because it can be fatal, any outbreak is often widely reported.

Bacteria that cause meningitis can live in the body and environment and remain harmless. However, when these bacteria get into the bloodstream, travel to the brain and spinal cord, and infect these regions, that's when the problem arises. The result is bacterial meningitis.

Bacterial meningitis causes behavioural changes and emotional disturbance including ADHD and learning difficulties. In children, it can lead to cognitive problems including low IQ, academic challenges and other issues with neurologically-based skills.

It's easy to confuse the early symptoms of meningitis with the flu. For this reason, parents need to stay alert to the key symptoms of meningitis – early treatment is key.

The hallmark symptoms are fever, headache, and neck stiffness. Confusion, disorientation, sensitivity to bright light, and drowsiness may be present. In some cases, there could be seizure and coma.

To reduce the risk of their child contracting meningitis, parents can follow these guidelines:

- Keep children away from infected people.
- Teach children good hygiene. Habits such as frequent washing of hands — especially after visits to public places and covering the mouth and nose when sneezing.
- Boost your child's immune system through a healthy lifestyle that incorporates a good diet, physical exercise, and mental relaxation.
- Teach children not to share eating utensils, toothbrushes, and other personal items with others.

Ear infections: Middle ear infection – otitis media (OM) is extremely common in childhood, affecting up to 80% of children before the age of 4 years. Studies demonstrate that repeated occurrences of OM can lead to long-term effects including a negative impact on cognitive and educational outcomes.

Williams and Jacobs, in their 2009 publication in the *Medical Journal of Australia* state that *"there is clear evidence that some patterns of the disease do predict long-term negative outcomes for speech and language."*

Linda Kreger Silverman, PhD, is an expert in giftedness and is the author of several publications. In a chapter in the book *Uniquely Gifted: Identifying and Meeting the Needs of Twice Exceptional Children,* she writes about OM and how chronic OM (more than nine ear infections before the age of three) can lead to problems with attention, listening skills, spelling, rote memorisation, and handwriting.

Further evidence of the impact of OM on IQ is presented in the *Archives of Disease in Childhood (2001).* Bennet et al analysed data pertaining to 1,000 children born in Dunedin, New Zealand, between 1 April 1972 and 31 March 1973. In their conclusion, the researchers state that middle ear disease in early years has a detrimental effect on reading ability, verbal IQ, and behaviour. The detrimental effect can persist into late childhood and early teens.

These are a few of the studies that declare that OM has a negative effect on cognition and achievement. However, other studies have yielded mixed results. Overall, researchers generally agree that a lot more research is required. Until research can categorically discount the effect of OM on IQ, parents should be conscious of persistent ear infections and their potential to damage IQ. Parents should not hesitate to seek medical advice as soon as there is any indication of an ear infection. As Dr Silverman states, *"Early diagnosis enables early intervention."*

BE AWARE OF HEALTH PROBLEMS THAT IMPACT IQ

Here are some measures that parents can take to ensure that any impact of health challenges that are known to adversely affect IQ are minimised:

- Do not smoke around children. Keep them away from environments where they will be exposed to second-hand smoke.

- If you notice that your child is stressed, work with them to identify and address the cause. In the meantime, use one or more of the many stress reduction techniques that can be found online to help them cope until the source of the stress is removed.

- Be aware of the key symptoms of diabetes, especially if there is family history of diabetes. Be vigilant with diet and physical exercise for your children and take them for regular medical check-ups.

- If there are there are cats in your home or work environment, or if your family eats partially-cooked or raw meat, it would be worthwhile for children (and parents) to be tested for toxoplasmosis.

- When travelling to countries where there is a risk of malaria, take precautions. Follow the ABCD code and be alert to possible infection.

- Learn the hallmark signs and symptoms of meningitis, and act quickly if you have any suspicions that you child has been infected.

- Be alert to persistent ear infections. The more frequent the occurrence in early childhood, the greater the risk of negative impact on IQ.

SECTION 4

ADDITIONAL STRATEGIES

20

Reading, Vocabulary, and IQ

"I would be most content if my children grew up to be the kind of people who think decorating consists mostly of building enough bookshelves."

Anna Quindlen, author and journalist

Reading is one of the few activities that allows a person to stimulate their mind, acquire new information, relax, enter a fantasy world, improve their communication skills, and much more all in one sitting. To instil in children a passion for reading is to bestow upon them a priceless gift — a gift that will last a lifetime. Reading is the gateway to knowledge and as research has shown, a route to greater intelligence.

How reading improves intelligence

In a study published in *Child Development* (2014), Scientists from the University of Edinburgh and King's College London discovered that reading and more specifically, enjoying reading, can lead to a real, measurable change in the brain and overall health. Beyond this, reading has a strong association with socioeconomic status (SES), education quality, and creativity. In other words, reading can improve general intelligence.

The researchers in this study focused on the links between reading ability and intelligence of 1,890 twins who were born in England and Wales and raised in the same family. The results showed that students who start early with reading scored higher on general intelligence tests, and read more over the years. Furthermore, those who read a lot enhanced their verbal and nonverbal intelligence as well — reading made them smarter.

Ritchie and Bates (2013) found that *"mathematics and reading ability both had substantial positive associations with adult SES, above and beyond the effects of SES at birth, and with other important factors, such as intelligence. "*

A paper published in *Perspectives on Psychological Science* titled *How to Make a Young Child Smarter: Evidence from the Database of Raising Intelligence* (2013) reported that up until the age of 4, reading to children in an interactive style raises their IQ by over 6 points. In interactive reading, the child is playing an active role in the reading and the adult encourages the child to expand on the story as much as possible.

The role of vocabulary

The role that vocabulary plays in intelligence is clearly indicated in a recent study published in the journal *Child Development* (2015). Researchers analysing data on 8,650 children found that 2-year-old children who arrived at kindergarten with larger oral vocabularies were better prepared academically and behaviourally than their peers. The children demonstrated greater achievement in reading and Maths, better self-regulation of behaviour, and fewer anxiety-related problem behaviours.

Paul Morgan, Associate Professor of Education at the Pennsylvania State University, who led the study stated, *"Our findings provide compelling evidence for oral vocabulary's theorized importance as a multifaceted contributor to children's early development ... Our findings are also consistent with prior work suggesting that parents who are stressed, overburdened, less engaged, and who experience less social support may talk, read, or otherwise interact with their children less frequently, resulting in their children acquiring smaller oral vocabularies."*

The researchers asserted that children starting kindergarten with higher maths and reading abilities have a higher probability of going to college, owning a home, getting married, and living in higher-income neighbourhoods when they are adults.

Dr Marion Blank, a world-renowned psychologist and expert on the development of literacy and language in children writes that *"Reading yields a snowball effect: the more one reads, the more one's vocabulary grows ... this is where the correlation between reading and intelligence is found".* Dr Blank's snowball effect is reinforced in the paper *What Reading Does for the Mind,* published in *Journal of Direct Instruction* (2001). In this paper, the authors emphasise the importance of reading volume on vocabulary development and point to statistical evidence indicating that reading volume is an especially effective way of increasing a child's vocabulary.

Dr Blank also asserts that it is not the words children learn in the early years such as car, run, girl, boy that make the difference. More advanced multi-syllable, harder words such as quality, escape, collapse, tranquil, and residence are the type of words that have a greater impact on intelligence. These are the types of words that should be taught sooner rather than later.

MAKE YOUR CHILD A READER

Reading is a passion, possibly one of the most important ones that parents should instil in children. The benefits beyond an increase in intelligence are numerous and far-reaching. Here are a few things you can do to start children on the path to becoming avid readers:

- Read interactively with your child — make it engaging and enjoyable. As you read, point out interesting pictures and ask questions. Use drama. Act out roles.

- Set aside time for nightly reading of good books. Not only can this build your child's reading abilities and intelligence, but it can also strengthen your relationship with your child.

- Have a good choice of books to choose from and let children choose their own books.

- For children above the age of 4, encourage reading of challenging selections. Good choices include events magazines, multi-content periodicals, and newspapers.

⚛ Avoid popular suspense fiction, as these books are not mentally stimulating. Instead, choose a classic novel or read concept books such as Richard Scarry's *Best First Book Ever* or DK Publishing's *My First Word Book* to your child.

⚛ Take the time to look up or explain the words your child does not know.

⚛ In addition to reading, some ways to help your child improve their vocabulary include:

- Teach harder words sooner rather than later.
- Play word games, such as board games or online games.
- Converse regularly with your child, engaging them in rich oral language.
- Relate known words to existing words.
- Improve your own vocabulary so that you can help your child learn new words.

21

Multiple Languages, Working Memory, and Intelligence

"Learning another language is not only learning different words for the same things, but learning another way to think about things."

Flora Lewis, American journalist

According to the *Psychology Today* (2010), more than half of the world's population is bilingual, that is, approximately 3.5 billion people. Being able to speak more than one language has many benefits, one of which is that it challenges the brain — thereby improving cognitive development.

Studies have established that when children learn a new language, it leads to strong thinking skills, and an improved ability to understand maths concepts more easily, use logical reasoning, and focus better. As well as this, children are able to interact with a more diverse group of people, which aids their social-emotional development. This chapter presents research demonstrating that being fluent in more than one language is an intelligence booster.

Working memory

Before we talk about multilingualism, let's talk about working memory. In the literature, there is little research that confirms a direct connection between IQ and fluency in multiple languages. There is, however, evidence to show that working memory is enhanced.

Why is working memory important? Well, for one thing, working memory and general intelligence are highly related (*Colom et al, Intelligence, 2008*). Also, good working memory is important for children because, as Professor Susan Gathercole and Dr Tracy Alloway state in *Understanding Working Memory, A Classroom Guide*

(2013), *"Many of the learning activities that children are engaged with in the classroom, whether related to reading, mathematics, science, or other areas of the curriculum, impose quite considerable burdens on working memory"*.

Prof. Gathercole and Dr Alloway go on to characterise children with poor working memory as:

- Reserved in group activities in the classroom.
- Forgetful of messages or instructions.
- Not seeing tasks through to completion.
- Frequently losing their place in complicated tasks, which they may then abandon.
- Making poor academic progress especially in reading and mathematics.

Working memory is important for tasks such as mental arithmetic and work that requires multi-tasking such as writing a meaningful sentence whilst trying to spell the words that are being written. Working memory is a mental workspace — a temporary holding space for information.

A small working memory is seen in children with many kinds of learning difficulties. A large working memory, on the other hand, increases the capacity to learn, understand, and participate — it is a prerequisite for exceptional performance in any complex environment. Dr Alloway even states that working memory is the new IQ.

The cognitive benefits of bilingualism and multilingualism

In 2010, researchers from Washington State University published an analysis of 63 studies on bilingualism. They to found that bilingual people outperform monolinguals in many activities related to attention, working memory and, abstract and symbolic skills.

Bilingual Brains – Smarter & Faster, published in *Psychology Today* (2011), highlighted the advantages of growing up in a bilingual household. In the article, the author writes that bilingual children demonstrate increased attentive focus and cognition compared to single language children.

On average, children with five to ten years of exposure to more than one language demonstrated higher scores in cognitive performance tests compared to monolinguals. The bilingual children displayed greater distraction resistance, attention focus, better decision-making, and improved judgment.

Küntay et al came to a similar conclusion when they measured the benefits of being bilingual in Turkish-Dutch children. Their work, published in the *Journal of Experimental Child Psychology* (2014), concluded that bilingualism enhances working memory and is associated with better verbal working memory performance. In the study, they examined a group of children at ages 4, 5, and 6. At age 6, they found that there was an overall advantage in working memory performance for the bilingual children over monolingual children.

Students in Florida who are bilingual scored 23-34 points higher on verbal and maths sections of the Florida standardized test than those who spoke only English. Dr Joanne H. Urrutia, Director of Florida's Bilingual Education and World Languages Department, suggests that the higher Maths scores may indicate bilingual students have advanced thinking skills and have developed a greater ability to think abstractly.

At the other end of the age spectrum, researchers from the Department of Psychology, National University of Singapore, found that even at the age of 6 months, infants who are exposed to more than one language have an advantage over babies in single language households. In the study published in *Child Development* (2014), they demonstrated that when repeatedly shown the same picture, bilingual babies get bored more quickly — they have a greater appetite for novel images. A baby's preference for novel stimuli and the speed at which it becomes bored have both been linked to performance in a range of cognitive areas. These are indicators of greater IQ and vocabulary later, during pre-school and school years.

Cerebral Cortex (2015) published a study demonstrating that multilingual people have more grey matter than those who only speak one language. Neuroimaging studies of the brain indicate that people with high IQ scores have significantly more grey matter than people with lower IQ scores (*Neuroimage, 2004 and 2003)*. So, it appears that as far as IQ is concerned, the more grey matter in the brain, the better.

The *Indiana Pathways Project Hoosier Briefs Issue 1* (2004) demonstrated the positive effect of bilingualism on SAT scores. The report presented data showing that the SAT scores of students who studied a foreign language for 1-3 years was, on average, 63 points higher than students who did not study a foreign language. The gap rose to 101 points when a foreign language was studied for 4 years.

A 2014 paper published in the *Annals of Neurology* described the results of re-testing the cognitive ability of 835 people who were originally tested in 1947 at the age of 11. Out of the 835 people who are now in their seventies, 262 knew at least two languages and they had cognitive abilities that were significantly better than the abilities than expectations based on their baseline test.

These are just a few of the studies supporting the case for encouraging children to learn a foreign language.

BECOME A MULTILINGUAL HOUSEHOLD

A second language (or more) is a valuable skill to acquire at any age. As well as having a positive effect on general intelligence, there are many other advantages of speaking more than one language. Here are some tips to set your child on the path to mastering several languages:

- Start off by helping your children to become bilingual. Later on, if they are willing, guide them to become fluent in as many languages as possible. Experts say that the more languages you learn, the easier it is to add more.

- If you live in a bilingual house, ensure that you continue to speak both languages so that your children become fluent in both languages.

- If you only speak one language, enrol your child on a language course.

- To make it more fun, join your children in learning a second language. That way, you learn a new language as well and you can practise together.

- Plan holidays to destinations where the new languages can be spoken. This will incentivise your child, and when on holiday, it will give them an opportunity to practise with native speakers.

- Watch foreign language TV channels together with your child.

- Use technologies such as "Suggestopedia" to make foreign language learning easier.

22

How Meditation Can Increase IQ

"Remember, meditation will bring you more and more intelligence, infinite intelligence, a radiant intelligence. Meditation will make you more alive and sensitive; your life will become richer."

Osho

There have literally been thousands of studies on meditation and mindfulness in which dozens of benefits, both mental and physical, have been identified. As a result of this research, there is now intense interest in meditation in school environments and high-tech hotspots such as Silicon Valley. Companies such as Google who recruit only the brightest people have developed meditation programs for their employees because they know that meditation helps the brain work better. Meditation helps the two hemispheres of the brain work synergistically. Boosting memory, increasing brain size and enhancing intelligence and IQ along the way.

Studies on meditation

The Scientific American (June 2014) reported on a study carried out by Adrienne Taren, a researcher studying mindfulness at the University of Pittsburgh. Taren carried out MRI scans on participants in an 8-week course of mindfulness practice. At the end of the 8 weeks, Taren noted that the brain's "fight or flight" centre (the amygdala) had shrank and its connection to the rest of the brain became weaker. In contrast to this, the part of the brain associated with higher order functions such as concentration, decision-making and awareness (the pre-frontal cortex) became thicker, and the connections between it and the rest of the brain became stronger. Taren also noted that the size of the changes in the brain correlated with the total number of hours of meditation practice a person had done.

Taren's research supports earlier research by Assistant Professor of Psychology at Harvard University Dr Sarah Lazar, who is the lead researcher on several studies on meditation and yoga. Using Magnetic Resonance Imagining (MRI), she was able to see that the brains of regular meditation and yoga practitioners were thicker in parts of the cerebral cortex linked to decision-making, memory, and attention.

Results from the study *Enhanced brain connectivity in long-term meditation practitioners*, which was published in *NeuroImage* (2011), revealed that changes observed in meditators involve large-scale networks, which include almost every part of the brain. Such large-scale cooperation within the brain improves brain functioning.

Hernandez et al, in *PLOS* (2016), also found large-scale changes in the brains of meditators. They investigated differences in grey matter volume between 23 experienced meditators and 23 non-meditators and found that the volume of grey matter across the whole brain was larger in meditators. Wilke et al *(Neuroimage, 2003)* found a strong correlation between IQ and volume of grey matter in the whole brain.

A study published in *Intelligence* (October 2001) presented results of three studies on 362 Taiwanese high school students which measured the effect of the consistent practice of Transcendental Meditation (TM) on cognitive ability. The children were required to meditate for 15–20 min twice a day for 6 to 12 months. Using seven standardized tests, Principal investigator and co-author Dr So Kam Tim measured a wide range of cognitive, emotional, and perceptual functions. The TM groups showed significant improvement in all seven areas compared to the control groups.

Additionally, the study showed that IQ as measured by the ability to reason in novel situations — "fluid intelligence" increased. Similarly, increased IQ was also indicated by a purely cognitive measure called "Inspection Time": improvement in basic aspects of intelligence, such as alertness and ability to focus, which are essential for learning. Improvements in the TM program groups were also found in practical intelligence, indicating increased non-intellectual abilities, such as optimism and the ability to work with others.

Dillbeck et al (1984) discovered a 9-point increase in IQ in a longitudinal study of students participating in a TM program. Cranson et al (1991) monitored 45 college students as they practiced TM over a two-year period. Their results indicated that the meditating students showed significant improvement on IQ-related measures of speed in processing complex information compared to 55 non-meditating students.

Shah et al (*Indian J Med Sci*, 2001), Singh, Sharma, and Talwar, (*Alternative Therapies*, 2012), Rosaen and Benn (2006) all found an increase in academic performance or IQ during their investigations into meditation. Additionally, the 10 young adolescents who were a part of the Rosean and Benn study also reported a state of restful alertness, increased self-reflection, and self-control.

Meditation facilitates faster neural communication and increased processing power by syncing both hemispheres of the brain. This was demonstrated in Alex Hankey's research published in *Evidence-based Complementary and Alternative Medicine* (January 2007). Hankey's research focused on the improvements observed in people who had been meditating for a long time. He noted a greater degree of whole brain function, greater awareness, improvements in sensory processing, and improved cognitive function.

When the logical left brain and creative right brain are in sync, deep thinking and problem solving becomes easier, creativity increases, and focus and concentration improve.

The benefits of meditation extend well beyond gains in intelligence. In America, some high schools in tough neighbourhoods now get pupils to do meditation rather than detention. The schools have seen a big drop-off in playground aggression, plus a rise in grades.

MEDITATION WILL MAKE YOUR CHILDREN MORE INTELLIGENT

Meditation has the potential to transform a child's life in many ways, beyond boosting brainpower, IQ, and memory. Encouraging children to meditate and adopt mindfulness practices techniques could help them to cope better with stress, perform better at school, and live healthier lives. Getting children to meditate, however, could be difficult. As any parent knows, children have a very short attention span! Here are some ways you could make a start:

- Start your children on the path to meditation as early in life as possible.

- Children are prone to copying the behaviour of their parents. Starting them on a meditation journey can be as simple as leading by example. If you currently don't meditate, you should start immediately. The benefits are compelling and undoubtable.

- Make meditation a part of the daily routine and then it will be easy to keep it up. It helps for children to either meditate right before they go to school or right before bed.

- Get professional help.

- Resources such as https://mindfulnessinschools.org are available to assist teachers and parents.

- Learning to meditate is not complex and there are many resources online. An excellent starting point is a beautiful 2-minute video called *How to Train Your Monkey Mind by Tibetan Buddhist Master Mingyur Riponche.* You can find this by searching online.

23

Brainwave Training and Neurofeedback

"Any man could, if he were so inclined, be the sculptor of his own brain."

Santiago Ramón y Cajal,
author of "Advice for a Young Investigator"

Our brain contains approximately 100 billion neurons and an estimated 100 trillion to 1,000 trillion synaptic connections. These neurons and synapses work together to send electrical signals to other neurons in the brain. The more efficiently neurons and synapses collaborate, the better the brain performs. Neurofeedback is exercise for the brain. It improves mental performance and intelligence by strengthening synaptic connections in the network of the brain. Neurofeedback is another technology that is being widely adopted by tech peak performers in the high-IQ, high-tech industries where superior intelligence is essential for competitive advantage.

What is neurofeedback?

Neurofeedback (also called neurotherapy, neurobiofeedback, or EEG biofeedback) is the direct training of brain function in which the brain learns to function more efficiently. Users observe the signals that their brains are emitting either visually on a screen or through sounds or both. They then learn how to use this feedback to consciously manipulate their thoughts and feelings to be more closely aligned with their desired goals. As they change their thoughts, they see and hear change on the monitors and they use this new feedback to make more changes, and so on. Eventually, the new patterns of thought become habitual and a potentially permanent change is created.

Dr Siegfried Othmer is an internationally recognised expert in the field of neurofeedback brainwave training. He defines neurofeedback as follows: *"The neurofeedback paradigm: by watching and listening to real-time multimedia representations of its own electrical activity, the brain can improve its functionality and even its structure."*

In *Development History of the Othmer Method: 1987 to 2016*, Dr Othmer reported that neurofeedback training brought benefits which included improvements memory-related tasks, logic handling abilities and reading comprehension. A follow-up with participants after one year also found improvements in creativity, self-concept, and concentration.

Neurofeedback feedback practitioners state that neurofeedback is very effective for children. They see significant benefits when working with young and flexible brains, before habits mature into traits in adulthood. In fact, as Dr Othmer states on his website, the initial impetus for him was the brain-training of their son for his seizure disorder, where the training was life-transforming. Indeed, some of the results reported by leading researchers show remarkable IQ improvements after neurofeedback training.

Neurofeedback and IQ

In 1996, Linden, Habib, and Radojevic published a paper titled *A Controlled Study of the Effects of EEG Biofeedback on Cognition and Learning.* Eighteen children diagnosed with ADD/ADHD and some with learning disabilities were IQ tested before and after neurofeedback. They reported an average 9-point improvement in IQ after neurofeedback.

An average 20-point improvement in IQ for 24 children was reported by M. A. Tansey in the *Australian Journal of Psychology* (December 1991). Similarly, in the journal *Applied Psychophysiology and Biofeedback* (1998), Thompson and Thompson reported an average 12-point improvement in IQ for 111 adults and children.

In the article *Development History of the Othmer Method 1987 to 2016*, Siegfried and Susan Othmer reported an average increase of 23 points for 85% of 726 students and 363 adults as a result of neurofeedback training. In a case study by Fleischman and Othmer published in *Journal of Neurotherapy* (2005), a pair of twins with mild developmental delay and some symptoms of ADHD showed IQ gains of 22 and 23 points following EEG biofeedback training. The improvements were maintained at three follow-ups over a 52-month period.

EXERCISE YOUR CHILD'S BRAIN WITH NEUROFEEDBACK

Neurofeedback training can be used to improve IQ. If you are interested in pursuing this approach, here are a few tips to get you started:

⚛ Chose a reputable neurofeedback training company. The best way to do this is through personal recommendations — somebody who has used the services of a company. Failing that, you can contact these organisations to find a practitioner:

- International Society for Neurofeedback & Research (ISNR) (https://www.isnr.org/).
- The Association for Applied Psychophysiology and Biofeedback (AAPB) https://www.aapb.org/.

Or you can search online for "neurofeedback training". Read the testimonials on the website and make sure the trainers are suitably qualified.

⚛ The first thing that reputable companies will do is an assessment. Following that, they will recommend a course of treatment. Costs will vary, so make sure that all the details are made clear during the first meeting.

⚛ Be aware that neurofeedback training will consist of a number of sessions, so it is wise to find a company that is relatively close to home. Some companies can do the training at home if that's more convenient for you.

24

Intelligence and Music

"If I were not a physicist, I would probably be a musician. I often think in music. I live my daydreams in music. I see my life in terms of music."

Albert Einstein, Physicist

Music is powerful. It heals, it soothes, it motivates. It is art, entertainment, pleasure, medicine for the heart and soul. It is an activity that involves using the whole brain. It is a catalyst for learning language, improving memory, and focusing attention as well as physical coordination and development. In this chapter, we look at the evidence supporting the theory that music can improve intelligence.

The Mozart effect – can listening to music increase IQ?

In the 1990s, the term "Mozart effect" was coined following research that reported a 9-point increase in the IQ score of subjects who listened to the music of Mozart. Whilst Mozart's music did raise IQ in the research undertaken in 1993 by Francis H. Rauscher, unfortunately, the effect was temporary and lasted only 10-15 minutes. Subsequent studies have confirmed that listening to music, in and of itself, does not affect IQ.

But that is not to say that listening to music is a complete waste of time when it comes to increasing IQ. Although it does not appear to lead to a permanent increase IQ, music can have an indirect impact on intelligence. For example, we know that vocabulary influences IQ as does learning foreign languages. There are technologies such as Suggestopedia that use music of a certain type to help people learn foreign languages and increase vocabulary faster and more easily than they could otherwise.

Also, music can help people to enter a meditative state — and meditation, as we know, positively influences IQ. These things apart, the only scientifically proven way to causally increase IQ through music is by learning to play an instrument.

The effect that learning to play music has on IQ

A 2004 study by E. Glenn Schellenberg of the University of Toronto at Mississauga demonstrated that nine months of weekly training in piano or voice increased the IQs of young students by nearly 3 points more than their untrained peers. Schellenberg says that there is a "dose-response association", which means that in general, the longer a child takes lessons, the higher the IQ and the better their performance in school.

In more recent work (2006), Schellenberg and his colleagues aimed to measure how IQ gains through music fared with age. They studied two groups of students: children from 6 to 11 years old and college freshmen aged between 16 and 25 who had taken music lessons in early childhood. In the case of the younger children, it was found that six years of lessons were associated with an increase in IQ of 7.5 points. However, the college freshmen, all of whom had stopped taking lessons and stopped playing regularly at the time of the study, demonstrated only a 2-point advantage in IQ. In other words, the strong gains in IQ tailed off later in life. It is not known whether this tail off would have persisted had the freshmen continued with their practice.

A 10-year study by James Catterall of UCLA involving 25,000 students established that test scores in standardized tests and in reading proficiency exams were improved by music-making. Similarly, *Profile of SAT and Achievement Test Takers, The College Board* (2001) reported that high school music students score higher on the maths and verbal portion of SAT compared to their peers.

When children learn to play a musical instrument, they learn how to make tunes and at the same time, boost motor and auditory skills, spatial learning skills, and memory. In addition, verbal memory, literacy, and verbal intelligence also benefit.

In 1997, Rauscher et al published the results of a study in *Neurological Research* in which 34 children received private piano keyboard lessons, 20 children received private computer lessons, and 24 children had no lessons. After six months, the children who received piano/keyboard training performed 34% higher on tests measuring spatial-temporal ability than the control group.

"Spatial-temporal reasoning," explains Dr Rauscher, *"is a very important component of proportional reasoning – understanding ratios and fractions. Good musicians...recognize patterns and familiar shapes. This type of thinking is very much like the way you think when you study mathematics [...] spatial-temporal reasoning allows one to make that link between music and mathematics."*

Is formal music training the only way to improve IQ?

Not all music training needs to be formal. Parents can start very early and in a playful way.

A 2015 carried out by the University of Queensland, Australia, found that even informal music activities with a toddler have an impact greater than that of reading to them. Through musical activities, a toddler benefits in multiple ways. They acquire positive social skills, learn attention regulation, and to a lesser extent, improve numeracy. The researchers stated that when an adult engages a child in playing music, the combination of face-to-face interaction, creativity, and sound results in learning that is reinforced by a positive, empathic emotional relationship.

Sylvain Moreno of York University conducted a study demonstrating that after only one month of music lessons in rhythm, pitch, melody, and voice, 90% of children between the ages of 4 and 6 had a significant increase in verbal intelligence. Moreno suggests that there was a "transfer effect" facilitated by the music training that increased the children's ability to understand words and explain their meaning.

Other research found that musically-trained children and adult women outperformed those without music training on verbal memory tests. The message is clear — to boost your verbal skills, try taking music lessons!

Can the genre of music that my children listen to affect IQ?

We know that there are IQ gains to be made — albeit transient — from listening to certain types of music, but are there types of music that damage intelligence? This is a question that many parents probably mull over when their child is listening to some deafeningly loud heavy metal or techno-rock.

The answer is that we don't know. A fun and interesting piece of informal research conducted by an enterprising 16-year old drew the attention of the press in 1997. David Merrill divided 72 mice into groups of 24. The first group — the control group — did not listen to any music. For 10 hours a day, the second group listened to Mozart and the third group listened to hard-rock. The mice were tested in a maze three times a week. Over time, David found that the control group mice managed reduce completion time by 5 minutes and the Mozart mice managed to take 8 ½ minutes off the completion time. The heavy rock mice, however, added 20 minutes to their time — 300% greater than their original. Unfortunately, David had to end the experiment prematurely because all the hard-rock mice killed each other!

On a more formal note, Gordon Shaw's work in 2000 indicated that rap and heavy metal negatively affect test performance — not IQ. Beyond this, there is little research investigating whether different types of music negatively affect intelligence.

USE MUSIC TO TUNE THE BRAIN

Music has universal appeal and the ability to powerfully affect brain states. You should make it a priority to introduce your children to music as early as possible in their childhood.

- Play musical games with your toddler. You could do something as simple as improvising a counting song or making new rhymes to a familiar song.

- Sign your children up for music lessons and encourage them to learn a musical instrument or vocal music.

- Singing classes will not only improve a child's intelligence, but it will also train them to breathe correctly. This will help to provide the brain with more oxygen.

- Music training and exposure to a wide variety of complex music such as Mozart is valuable because it can increase a child's IQ score and because it contributes in more intangible ways to a child's development.

25

Image Streaming

"Image-Streaming can powerfully help you to: solve problems; discover answers; profoundly accelerate learning; inform you about all sorts of aspects of your world and those around you and about yourself; and even accelerate and improve your reading."

Win Wenger, PhD, researcher, author, and teacher

Image streaming is one of those off-grid yet extremely interesting techniques that deserves more scientific investigation than it has received. It is a simple technique that is easily applied across all age groups and holds the promise of significant IQ gains if practised regularly.

Image streaming is a technique developed by Win Wenger PhD, author of the books *The Einstein Factor and How to Increase Your Intelligence*. It is a method of brain training that results in a permanent increase in IQ. According to Dr Wenger, *"Where participants have participated to 50 hours, 40 points IQ gain appear and we have not yet found any point where the benefits might start tailing off."*

The method is very simple and consists of closing your eyes and describing, out loud, the images that appear in your mind. You need an external focus to describe your images to. This external focus can be a person or a recording device. It doesn't matter about the quality or clarity of the image that is seen in the mind's eye. The key is to examine and describe it aloud, in as rich detail as possible, even if you feel at first that you are "forcing" or "faking" some of it. Over time, images will become rich and vivid.

Dr Wenger has dedicated most of his life to finding ways to increase intelligence. On his website, he describes in detail how the method can be applied to children. The article can be found by searching using the search term: "image streaming for young children".

In the article, he states that, "*The impact of Image Streaming in a young child, upon language, brain, perception, understanding, thoughtfulness, and apparent intelligence is so great and so immediate, that to see those immediate effects has been, time and again, this writer's most rewarding experience ever!*"

The potential gains from image streaming are significant and well worth investigating. In 1988 Charles P. Reinert, a professor at Southwest State University, Minnesota, used the image streaming protocol to investigate whether he could increase the IQ of students with an average IQ. The method he used is as follows:

1) Find someone to listen as you describe the images that come from your stream of consciousness, or if you prefer, record yourself describing the images.

2) Sit comfortably. Sitting is preferred over lying down to stop you going to sleep.

3) Close your eyes and look into the blackness.

4) Start describing, aloud, using present tense: "I see…" followed by anything that arises. For example, various colours, lines, images, lights, shapes, and forms may appear. The description doesn't have to be precise and you can exaggerate, enhance, and embellish whatever way you choose. Remember to describe out loud, and as you are describing, try to use as many senses as you can (sight, sound, touch, smell, taste.)

5) Do this for 10 minutes initially and then move to 15-20 minutes.

Over a duration of 40 hours, Reinert's team measured a **20-point increase in IQs.** In addition to IQ gains, creativity, vivid mental imagery, cross-hemispheric communications, and verbal fluency all improved.

At the end of his study, Professor Reinert stated he remained "*very impressed with not only the quantitative improvement, which seems to accompany the image streaming process, but also its ease of use. I have yet to work with a student who, when using proper technique, was unable to 'get pictures'. Some are of course much better at the process than others, but it seems possible, and relatively easy, for all to successfully use this technique.*"

Although there are no further empirical scientific studies available, Dr Wenger's image streaming testimonials include many who have tried and benefitted from this approach.

IMAGE STREAMING IS A FUN AND EASY WAY TO INCREASE IQ

Image streaming is a proven and relatively rapid way of greatly increasing IQ. It is an easy way to improve IQ, which comes with other benefits.

⚛ Dr Wenger recommends that the best way to teach image streaming to a child is to first learn it yourself. If you are fairly smooth and practiced with your own image streaming, then it will be much easier to teach the method to your children.

⚛ When you are comfortable with your own image streaming and you are ready to start teaching it to your children, Dr Wenger suggests proceeding as follows:

- Say something like this to your child (substitute your child's name for Mary):

  "Mary, did you know that even when we are awake we have dreams going on inside us? Now, I am going to close my eyes and tell you what I can see... I see... two big trees... they are very tall... a bit like the trees that we saw in the park on Sunday. Because it's windy, I can see the branches moving and I can hear the leaves rustling. In one of the trees, I see a squirrel standing on a branch. It is standing up on its back legs and looking at me. It looks so cute. It's decided to run down the tree and onto the green grass just in front of me... I think it wants to come to me but just as it's about to come forward, a dog comes running towards us. It's a beautiful big white dog with black spots. I think the dog wants to play but the squirrel is scared and runs up the other tree... the dog looks puzzled."

- What you have just recited to Mary is your image stream. This shows Mary how to do it. Now you give Mary a chance by saying something along the lines of "Okay, now, when you close your eyes, tell me what you see there..."

⚛ Search for "image streaming for young children" to find Win Wenger's full instructions for image streaming.

26

Television

"I find television very educating. Every time somebody turns on the set,
I go into the other room and read a book."

Groucho Marx, comedian and film star

In most households of developed nations, the television is a central feature in their house. It is something that many families gather around and something that children are exposed to on an almost daily basis from birth. There is no doubt that television has a good side — it can be both educational and entertaining. However, the reverse is also true — it has the potential to have a negative effect on children in many ways. In this chapter, we look at the pros and cons of TV in relation to intelligence.

The negative effects of TV

Many parents allow their infants and toddlers to watch TV and videos alone because they believe that some programs improve their child's intelligence. However, several studies prove that this is not always the case.

The most effective way for children to watch educational programs is with a parent or other caregiver. The parent's presence and interaction is particularly important during early childhood because, as research scientist Yalda T. Uhls of the Children's Digital Media Center wrote in a BBC News article, *"Without social interactions, screens at young ages don't teach anything"*. According to Uhls, children who are under 2 years of age are not capable of understanding that the world that they see on the TV screen is supposed to correspond to the real world. As a result, they find it difficult to translate what they see into real life — they need parents and caregivers to interact with them to help them understand.

In a 2007 study published in *The Journal of Pediatrics* (2007), 1008 parents of children aged between 2 to 24 months were surveyed about their interactions with their children, the child and parent demographics, and the types TV and DVD/video programs that the child viewed. Parents were also asked to fill in a Communicative Development Inventory (CDI) form — a form that records a child's abilities in early language including vocabulary and grammar. The CDI form is a useful measure of intelligence because of the high correlation between vocabulary and intelligence.

The study revealed that for infants aged between 8 and 16 months, every hour in a day that a child watched baby DVDs or videos, a 16.99-point decrease in CDI score was registered. Based on these results, the researchers arrived at the conclusion that watching baby DVDs/videos in early years hinders language development.

In 2013, neuroscientist Hikaru Takeuchi had similar findings for older children. Takeuchi imaged the brains of 290 children aged between 5 and 18 and noted their TV viewing habits. He discovered that the more TV children watched, the lower their verbal IQ scores. A few years later, in a follow-up study involving 235 of the original 290 children, he saw a further decline in verbal IQ.

Further evidence that watching TV in the early years hinders some facets of a child's development comes from a 2004 study published by Zimmerman and Christakis. They found that children who watched the greatest amount of TV up to the age of 3 performed the worst on Mathematics and reading tests at the ages of 6 and 7. Hancox et al (2005) investigated the long-term impact of watching too much TV in a study of 1,000 New Zealand children. They found that TV viewing time between the ages of 5-11 and 13-15 correlated to leaving school early and not attaining a university degree.

As well as the direct developmental issues just described, research has unearthed other negative factors associated with TV. Namely, TV can lead to sleep problems and influence children to start smoking and drinking alcohol during adolescence — all of which negatively affect IQ.

Lastly, there is evidence that watching TV in the early years forms a habit that persists into the later years of childhood — TV can become addictive.

Evidence in favour of TV

Despite the evidence citing the negative effects of TV, there are a few studies indicating that under some circumstances, TV can aid in a child's intellectual development.

Although Zimmerman and Christakis reported that children younger than 3 were adversely affected by TV, they also found that children aged 3 to 5 **did** derive some benefit from TV. Their theory is that at the time of the study, very few educational programs for under-3s were broadcast in the United States. However, there were a large number of educational programs such as *Sesame Street*, which were targeted at the 3-5 age group. They reasoned that this could be why some benefit was seen in the older group.

In more recent research, a 2013 study carried out at the University of London concluded that 3-year-old children who watched three or more hours of TV a day were three months ahead of their peers who watched less than an hour a day. However, the researchers stated that these positive results were only seen for less educated mothers. The report's lead author Dr Alice Sullivan, Senior Academic at the University's Institute of Education, said that in these instances, TV *"may also help expose some children to a broader vocabulary than they get at home"*.

LIMIT THE AMOUNT OF TV YOUR CHILDREN WATCH

Whilst much more research needs to be undertaken to evaluate the effects of TV on children's IQs, most of the research to date indicates that watching TV does more harm than good when it comes to intelligence. For one thing, more time spent sitting on the couch watching TV means less time spent in physical activity, being out in nature, reading, and interacting with friends. This lack of physical activity and intellectual pursuits has obvious physical and cognitive consequences.

❀ In 2016, the American Academy of Pediatrics issued new guidelines for children's media use. In those guidelines, they recommended the following constraints. You may choose to implement a few or all of them:

Age range	Viewing advice
0-18 months	No screen time except video-chatting.
18-24 months	Only high-quality programming. To be watched with parents who can then help them to understand what they are watching.
2-5 years	Limit to 1 hour of high-quality programs per day. To be watched with parents to help children understand the content and how it is relevant to the world around them.
6 and older	Consistent limits on media time, type, and content. Ensure that media does not take the place of adequate sleep, physical activity, and other behaviours essential to health.
All	Schedule media-free times together, such as dinner or driving, and create some media-free locations at home, such as bedrooms.

❀ Resist the temptation to habitually use TV as a way of keeping your children busy so that you pursue other activities.

❀ Consider following in the footsteps of many parents who have discarded their TV.

27

Video Games

"Games are transforming the brains of people who play them in largely positive ways."

Jane McGonigal, American game designer and author

According to Newzoo, a leading provider of market intelligence, the global video games market reached $99.6 billion in 2016. Video games are big business! Although players of all ages love video games, many parents don't share this love. Many parents feel that in moderation, games are a fun way to pass time, but worry that they probably do little — if anything — to make a person smarter and improve their IQ. The rise of video games is attracting researchers to study the effects of video gaming on gamers.

How video games can affect IQ

Recent research is disproving what many parents think about video games being purely a way to pass time.

A study that was published in *Social Psychiatry and Psychiatric Epidemiology*, (2016), used data from a Pan-European project to see how time spent on video games affects young children. The analysis revealed that, compared to non-gamers, the most enthusiastic gamers in this group of 6 to 11 year olds were 1.75 more likely to demonstrate high intellectual functioning and 1.88 times as likely to exhibit high overall school performance. Unfortunately, this doesn't necessarily mean that the more video games that your children play, the more intelligent they will become — researchers cautioned against unrestrained gaming. However, it does indicate that if your child is a keen gamer, they are probably very intelligent.

In July 2016, *Scientific American* published *The Brain Boosting Power of Video Games*. In the article, the authors stated that preconceptions of video gamers as being impulsive and easily distracted is outdated. What research actually demonstrates is that both children and adults who immerse themselves in the fantasy world of video games gain significant cognitive benefits.

Many experiments performed in the past few years have indicated that several aspects of brain function can be improved through gaming. These include: memory, problem solving skills, spatial reasoning, strategic planning and attention span. Even social skills can receive a boost.

In 2014, scientists from the Max Planck Institute for Human Development and Charite University Medicine measured the brain volume of a group of people. Half of the group were then asked to play Super Mario 64 for a minimum of 30 minutes per day for two months whilst the other half played no games. After the two-month period, when the brain volume of each participant was re-measured, researchers found a significant increase in grey matter of the people who played the game. The areas of the brain that saw the most growth were the ones that control spatial navigation, strategic planning, and working memory. There was no increase in grey matter of the control group.

In 2012, Dr Tracy Alloway published the results of a study in which she provided a game that targeted the memory centres of the brain to over 600 children aged six to sixteen. The game and had 30 levels of ascending difficulty. Players were required to remember various patterns and numbers as they flashed on a screen so that they could use them in a subsequent task. Over an eight-week period, gamers had to play four times a week for 15 minutes.

Results indicated that for 90% of the students who took part in the experiment, there was a significant improvement in their mathematical and verbal problem-solving skills. Also, their post-training verbal IQ increased by 7 points, and, at the 8-month follow-up, the IQ score increased by almost 11 points.

Researchers from Queen Mary University of London and the University College of London conducted a which set out to measure the effect of different types of games on cognitive flexibility. Half of a group of 72 volunteers selected for the study played StarCraft – a real time military strategy game *StarCraft* whilst the other half played *The*

Sims - a game that doesn't require any military tactics or strategy. The results, published in the journal *PLOS One (2013)* showed that in tests of cognitive flexibility, *StarCraft* players were faster and more accurate than players of *The Sims*.

> *Not all video games are created equal. Some games have a positive effect on cognitive functions whilst others have no effect. To maximise the brain-building benefits of games, parents should identify and select games that develop strategic planning and problem-solving skills.*

Which types of games help to develop the brain?

Puzzle games and games that require jumping from around, avoiding missiles, negotiating obstacles can improve brain function and IQ because they rely on problem-solving, memory, spatial reasoning, and attention to detail. A good example is *Angry Birds*.

Role playing games are games in which the player adopts the role of a character. They can improve problem-solving, strategy, logic, and reasoning skills. These games usually focus on a players' choices, options offered through dialogues, and the consequences of what the player has chosen to do. Another advantage of these games is that, because they are frequently faced with difficult choices that have consequences, players can practice social skills such as empathy and test their moral principles. One example of a famous role play game is *Final Fantasy*.

Real-time strategy games use strategy and planning skills to complete a task. The usual aim is to conquer the enemy - working alone or as part of a team. This genre of games improves planning, multitasking, prioritisation skills and, because the games are real time, they also teach people how to adapt to change. An example of a real-time strategy game is *StarCraft II*.

With all the research indicating that video games can have academic benefits, some schools are changing the traditional school setup in favour of a game-based approach. At New York's Quest to Learn middle school, specialized games are brought into the classroom. An article in the *Huffington Post* (December 2015) reports that students at the school performed better in English and Maths scores than their traditionally schooled peers. The article states that *"In 2013, 56 percent of Quest middle-school students scored better than the citywide average on the state standardized English Language Arts exams, and 43 percent exceeded the citywide average for math."*

What about the negatives associated with video games?

Despite the positives, there are still some things to watch out for when it comes to gaming. As with any fun activity, it is easy to become so engrossed in a game that it starts to negatively affect school and social activities. Being stuck to a console takes away time from more creative pursuits such as music and art. In addition, physical exercise may be reduced if a child spends most of their time seated playing games.

Online games can connect children with other gamers across time zones, making it easy for gamers to become so engrossed in games that they lose track of time and sacrifice sleep in order to continue playing. More concerning than sleep deprivation is the fact that through online games, children are interacting with complete strangers. The potential for cyber bullying, grooming, and exploitation is huge. For this reason, this type of gaming requires more policing and tighter regulation by parents.

Another concern amongst parents, legislators, and psychologists is that violence in games negatively affects children. The results of a 2010 meta-analysis of 136 research papers by Anderson and colleagues add weight to these concerns. The results show that playing violent video games leads to an increase in the likelihood of physically aggressive behaviour, aggressive thinking, aggressive affect, and physiological arousal.

SOME VIDEO GAMES CAN INCREASE IQ

Research has established that certain video games can be useful in enhancing IQ. However, there are some points that parents need to consider:

⚛ Regulate gaming to ensure that other important activities such as socialising, reading, sports, and sleep are not compromised.

⚛ Take extra care when children are playing online. Monitor conversations, and keep a lookout for behaviour that is associated with grooming, exploitation, or bullying such as the following:

- Being very secretive online and offline.
- Going to unusual places to meet friends.
- Having new things such as clothes or gadgets that can't be explained.
- Giving away or "losing" clothes and gadgets.
- Suddenly talking about and justifying the use of drugs and alcohol.

⚛ Parents need to ensure that games are age-appropriate and challenge the player in a way that boosts IQ.

⚛ Overtly violent games and games with inappropriate content should be avoided, especially for young children:

- Each game has an age rating that you can use as the first check for suitability.
- Go online to read reviews of games. A useful site is www.commonsensemedia.com.
- Spend a short time watching your child playing the game.
- If the game is unsuitable, return it.

CONCLUSION

The preceding 27 chapters in this book list many ways that IQ can be influenced — in an upward or downward direction. To maximise your child's IQ, do the things that increase IQ and stop doing the things that decrease IQ. Take an incremental approach — one step at a time. Have fun along the way and you'll find that as you help your child develop, the parent-child bond will also get stronger.

Parenting is sometimes challenging, but more often, it is utterly rewarding. Knowing that you have enabled your children to realise their potential and make full use of their innate intelligence is, in many ways, so much more satisfying than just materially providing for them.

Join your children on the journey and increase your IQ too. Even better — get the whole family involved! Many of the strategies presented in this book can be integrated into a healthy lifestyle and have the potential to benefit the whole family. After all, there is nothing to lose and much to gain.

Enjoy the journey and good luck!

Jagir S. Reehal

For additional useful information, news about related products and to contact the author visit www.thesuccessfulkid.com

www.ingramcontent.com/pod-product-compliance
Lightning Source LLC
Chambersburg PA
CBHW031958040426
42448CB00006B/411